**Longitudinal Endosonography
Atlas and Manual
for Use in the Upper Gastrointestinal Tract**

T. Rösch, U. Will, K.J. Chang (Editors)

Springer

Berlin
Heidelberg
New York
Barcelona
Hong Kong
London
Milan
Paris
Singapore
Tokyo

T. Rösch • U. Will
K.J. Chang (Editors)

Longitudinal Endosonography

**Atlas and Manual
for Use in the
Upper Gastrointestinal Tract**

With 320 Figures

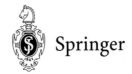

Springer

Rösch, T.
2. Medizinische Klinik
Klinikum Rechts der Isar der TU München
Ismaninger Strasse 22
D-81675 München, Germany
Tel.: +49-89-4140-4772; Fax: +89-4140-4872;
e-mail: Thomas.Roesch@lrz.tu-muenchen.de

Will, U.
Klinik für Innere Medizin I
Friedrich-Schiller-Universität Jena
Erlanger Allee 101
D-07747 Jena, Germany
Tel. +49-3641-939-108; Fax.: +49-3641-939-291
e-mail: WILL@polkim.med.uni-jena.de

Chang, K.J.
UCI Medical Center
Chao Family Comprehensive Cancer Center
Gastrointestinal Oncology
101, The City Drive, Bldg. 23, Rt. 81, Rm. 330
Orange, C92668, USA
(e-mail: kchang@uci.edu)

ISBN 3-540-65586-7
Springer-Verlag Berlin Heidelberg New York

Die Deutsche Bibliothek – CIP-Einheitsaufnahme
Longitudinal endosonography: atlas and manual for use in the upper gastrointestinal tract/Th. Rösch ... (ed.). – Berlin; Heidelberg; New York; Barcelona; Budapest; Hong Kong; London; Milan; Paris; Singapore; Tokyo: Springer, 2001
   ISBN 3-540-65586-7

Springer-Verlag Berlin Heidelberg New York a member of BertelsmannSpringer Science+Business Media GmbH

http://www.springer.de

© Springer-Verlag Berlin Heidelberg 2001
Printed in Germany

The use of general descriptive names, registered names, trademarks, etc. in this publication does not imply, even in the absence of a specific statement, that such names are exempt from the relevant protective laws and regulations and therefore free for general use.

Product liability: The publishers cannot guarantee the accuracy of any information about the application of operative techniques and medications contained in this book. In every individual case the user must check such information by consulting the relevant literature.

Cover design: design & production, Heidelberg
Printing and bookbinding: Stürtz AG, Würzburg

SPIN: 10702646   18/3130 – 5 4 3 2 1 0
Printed on acid-free paper

Preface

Endoscopic ultrasonography is now about 20 years old. It has significantly extended our diagnostic possibilities in gastroenterology. Due to its unique diagnostic capability that allows high resolution imaging of the GI wall and neighbouring organs, more information can be obtained about the local extent and growth of gastrointestinal and pancreatobiliary tumors. In addition, EUS has substantially contributed to the diagnosis of small pancreatic exocrine and endocrine tumors as well as submucosal gastrointestinal lesions. A large body of literature has accumulated, that shows good to excellent accuracy rates of EUS in these indications. These indications have been established by numerous papers and consensus statements of endoscopic societies. The more recent papers, concentrating on the influence of EUS on outcome and on cost effectiveness, have also shown a distinct role of this procedure in diagnostic gastroenterology.

There are, however, also limitations of EUS. These mainly lie in the limited ability to differentiate between benign and malignant lesions. One way to solve these problems, at least partially, has been the introduction of EUS guided fine needle puncture. To perform this safely and effectively, longitudinal scanning echo-endoscopes were developed. Previously available radially scanning instruments are considered not as suitable for this purpose. Since most papers on diagnostic EUS have been published with respect to the radial scanner, there is little experience in the literature on the accuracy of linear scanning in the classical indications of EUS. The few comparative studies suggest, that both instruments may be equivalent regarding the standard applications of EUS. However, there is little basic information about linear anatomy whereas the number of publications on EUS guided fine needle puncture is still growing.

The present book will hopefully serve as a tool to endosonographers, who are working exclusively with the longitudinal scanners. The anatomy section correlates the endosonographic images with cross-sectional anatomy. The whole spectrum of pathological findings is then presented in detail with some tips and tricks. Finally, EUS guided puncture and the recent field of EUS-related therapy are covered in detail.

We are extremely grateful to our coauthors, who have invested enormous work into this project. The pictures were collected from a large pool during two conferences of the participating authors and reviewed by the group. Our special thanks go to Dr. Raman Muthusamy for his tremendous effort in clarifying the EUS terminology. Mr. Holger Frey from Hitachi Ultrasound did a tremendous job in putting the pictures into an electronic format. We would like to convey special thanks from the authors to him. The present book is supported by Hitachi Ultrasound, based on an initiative by Mr. Karl-Heinz Pelster, and the Pentax Company. It is for this reason that only images produced by Pentax/Hitachi are included. The same anatomic principles, however, also apply to other longitudinal instruments. With Springer-Verlag as our publisher, we are be confident that the widespread distribution of this book as an educational tool is guaranteed. We also thank Mr. Thomas Günther, from Springer, for his oversight and organization.

On behalf of the authors, we hope that this book will be of practical help to the users of linear echo-endoscopes, showing the advantages and limitations of longitudinal EUS and being instructive for performing EUS guided fine needle puncture.

Thomas Rösch
Uwe Will
Kenneth J. Chang

Contents

Contributors

Burmester, E.
Städtisches Krankenhaus Süd
Zentrum Innere Medizin
Kronsforder Allee 71-73
D-23560 Lübeck, Germany
Tel.: +49-451-5851405; Fax:+49-451-5851234
e-mail: e.burmester@khs.de

Chang, K.J.
UCI Medical Center
Chao Family Comprehensive Cancer Center
Gastrointestinal Oncology
101, The City Drive, Bldg. 23, Rt. 81, Rm. 330
Orange, C92668, USA
e-mail: kchang@uci.edu

Chen, Y.K.
Division of Gastroenterology & Hepatology
University of Colorado Health Sciences Center
Campus Box B-158
4200 East Ninth Avenue
Denver, CO 80262
Tel (303)-315-7132;
Fax (303)-372-4056; efax (781)-623-8587
e-mail: Yang.Chen@UCHSC.edu

Erk, J.-U.
Abt. Innere Medizin, Diakonissenkrankenhaus
Holzhofgasse 29
D-01099 Dresden, Germany
Tel.: +49-351-8101-664; Fax: +49-351-8101-658

Greiner, L.
Klinikum Wuppertal, Medizinische Klinik 2
Abt. Gastroenterologie und Hepatologie
Heusnerstrasse 40
D-42283 Wuppertal, Germany
Tel.: +49-202-896-2248; Fax: +49-202-896-2740

Jacobsen, G.-K.
Copenhagen University Hospital Gentofte
Dept. of Pathology
DK-2900 Hellerup, Danmark
Tel.: +45-3-977-3977; Fax: +45-3-977-7679

Jakobeit, C.
Johanniter-Krankenhaus, Innere Medizin
Siepenstrasse 33
D-42477 Radevormwald, Germany
Tel.: +49-2195-600-228; Fax: +49-2195-600-157

Janssen, J.
Klinikum Wuppertal, Medizinische Klinik 2
Abt. Gastroenterologie und Hepatologie
Heusnerstrasse 40
D-42283 Wuppertal, Germany
Tel.: +49-202-896-2610; Fax: +49-202-896-2740;
e-mail: jjanssen@klinikum-wuppertal.de

Kann, P.
Klinik und Poliklinik Innere Medizin
Schwerpunkt Endokrinologie
und Stoffwechselkrankheiten
Klinikum der Johannes-Gutenberg-
Universität Mainz
D-55101 Mainz, Germany
Tel.: +49-6131-17-6844; Fax: +49-6131-17-5506;
e-mail: pkann@mail.uni-mainz.de

Muthusamy, V.R.
Division of Gastroenterology
University of California
San Francisco
Box 0535, S-357
513 Parnassus Avenue
San Francisco, CA 94143
USA

Plies, W.
Product-Manager
Hitachi Ultrasound GmbH
Kreuzberger Ring 21
D-65205 Wiesbaden, Germany
Tel.: +49-611-973220; Fax: +49-611-9732210;
e-mail: w.plies@hitachi-ultrasound.com

Rösch, T.
2. Medizinische Klinik
Klinikum Rechts der Isar der TU München
Ismaninger Strasse 22
D-81675 München, Germany
Tel.: +49-89-4140-4772; Fax: +89-4140-4872;
e-mail: thomas.roesch@lrz.tu-muenchen.de

Seifert, H.
Medizinische Klinik II, Endoskopie,
Abteilung für Gastroenterologie
Johann-Wolfgang-Goethe-Universität
Theodor-Stern-Kai 7
D-60590 Frankfurt / Main, Germany
Tel.: +49-69-6301-5333, Fax: +49-69-6301-6247
e-mail: seifert@em.uni-frankfurt.de

Stief, M.
European Sales/Marketing Manager
Pentax GmbH
Julius-Vosseler-Strasse 104
D-22527 Hamburg, Germany
Tel.: +49-40-5619-2148; Fax: +49-40-560-4213
e-mail: medica@pentax.de

Vilmann, P.
Copenhagen University Hospital, Gentofte
Dept. of Surgical Gastrointesterology
DK-2900 Hellerup, Danmark
Tel.: +45-3-9777-950; Fax: +45-3-9777-679
e-mail: pevi@gentehoftehosp.khamt.dk

Welp, L.
Johanniter-Krankenhaus, Innere Medizin
Siepenstrasse 33
D-42477 Radevormwald, Germany
Tel.: +49-2195-600-228, Fax: +49-2195-600-157

Will, U.
Klinik für Innere Medizin I
Friedrich-Schiller-Universität Jena
Erlanger Allee 101
D-07747 Jena, Germany
Tel.: +49-3641-939-108; Fax: +49-3641-939-291
e-mail: WILL@polkim.med.uni-jena.de

Wittenberg, M.
Prosper-Hospital
Akademisches Lehrkrankenhaus
der Ruhr-Universität Bochum
Medizinische Klinik
Mühlenstrasse 27
D-45659 Recklinghausen, Germany
Tel.: +49-2361-540, Fax: +49-2361-542-696
e-mail: markus.wittenberg@ruhr-uni-bochum.de

PART 1

Basic Principles

W. Plies · M. Stief

CHAPTER 1
Basic Principles and Technology

Ultrasound was introduced as a new tool in medical diagnosis in 1947. This technology is based on transmission of high-frequency sound waves or pressure waves through a medium. Unlike electromagnetic waves, sound waves cannot be transmitted through a vacuum or gas.

The piezo-electrical effect causes a conversion from electrical to mechanical energy by applying a voltage to a transducer element which results in the emission of sound waves. The sound waves produced follow the physical laws that apply to optics; namely reflection and refraction. Presently, the frequencies of sound waves utilized for medical diagnostic applications ranges from 1 MHz up to 20 MHz.

The latest research on diagnostic ultrasound is aimed at utilizing even higher frequencies, as axial resolution directly correlates with wavelength. The wavelength is inversely proportional to the frequency. However, penetration of higher frequency ultrasound waves is limited by the dampening factor (expressed in decibels per cm per megahertz), requiring lower frequencies for deeper penetration.

Ultrasound travels in human soft tissue with an average velocity of 1540 m/s. Ultrasound units are calibrated to this value, allowing distance measurements in the tomographic image.

Processing of the reflected echoes results in a B-Mode (Brigtness Mode) image with a grayscale, with bright pixels representing strong echoes and darker pixels representing weaker echoes.

When an ultrasonic wave encounters a moving target, the frequency of the echo will be sligthly altered. This is explained by the Doppler effect. In practice this effect is applied to visualize the blood flow by generating a spectral waveform quite similar to an ECG tracing. Using the same basic Doppler principle, color images can be generated in real-time showing vessels and their blood flow in B-Mode images.

Technical Aspects on Endosonography

Ultrasound scanning under endoscopic guidance, called Endoscopic Ultrasound (EUS), is one of the more recent applications of diagnostic ultrasound. EUS use has rapidly expanded since its first clinical utilization starting around 1980. Much earlier, in 1957, a first attempt using blind endoscopic ultrasound was done by Wild and Reid using a mechanically rotating scanner in the rectum. Shortly thereafter, endosonography was successfully used in other endocavity applications such as transvaginal and transesophageal examinations. The availability of more sophisticated transducers and probes led to an increasing use of endosonography, generating clinically relevant diagnostic information in gastroenterology, obstetrics/gynecology, urology, and cardiology.

The first flexible instruments were based on longitudinal scanning technique using electronic curved array transducers and the complementary radial scanning technique with mechanical transducers (Fig. 1.1).

Today, a range of instruments is available and improvements are being made with respect to

- the size and frequency of transducers in order to achieve the highest resolution and sufficient penetration
- the efficiency of ultrasound processors used to visualize the morphology of gastrointestinal structures in real-time
- the maneuverability and thickness of the rigid distal part as well as the insertion tube, giving efficient access to lesions and lessening patient discomfort
- endoscopic image quality comparable to that available in conventional flexible endoscopes

The Mechanical Radial Scanner

This ultrasound endoscope is equipped with side viewing optics and a distally placed mechanically rotating scanning transducer. Perpendicular to the axis of the insertion tube the ultrasonic scan field is generated by a single crystal element undergoing 360 degree rotation. Due to the circumferential visualization of luminal structures and adjacent organs, the orientation is considered easier compared with the longitudinal approach of the curved linear array scanner (Fig. 1.1). The continuous rotation is generated by an acoustic mirror connected to both a flexible drive shaft and a motor placed outside on the control body of the instrument. The fiber optics and steering controls function in the same way as in conventional endoscopes. To reduce mechanical damage, the motor drive must be stopped during insertion and removal of the probe. As with all side or oblique viewing optics, it is advisable to carefully check the lumen for any obstruction and not forcefully traverse a stenosis which bears the risk of perforation. Most radial scanning instruments also include a working channel mainly used for irrigation and suction. However, due to the 90° offset between the ultrasonic field and direction of the working channel, an ultrasound guided puncture cannot be safely performed. This is because there is no visual control of the needle tip during advancement of the needle (Fig 1.2).

The ultrasonic signal is generated by a pulsating unit feeding the single element crystal, and the reflecting echoes are received and amplified in the processor unit. Here, the signal information of each radial geometric scanning line is positioned according to the 360 degree encoding system in the mechanical drive unit. The scan converter transfers the echo information into a sequence of images which are displayed on a TV monitor. Since this book concentrates on longitudinal EUS. further instrument details are not given.

The Longitudinal Convex Array Scanner

The Pentax-Hitachi FG 32 UA unit was introduced 1991. This instrument consists of an oblique forward viewing fiberoptics gastroscope with a curved linear array transducer mounted in front of the lens. The

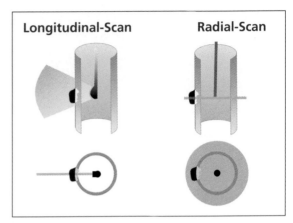

Fig. 1.1

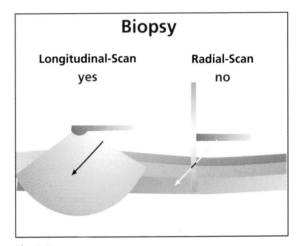

Fig. 1.2

transducer is based on high density technology with 192 elements. The fiberoptic view coincides with the ultrasound scanning plane, which allows simultaneous observation of luminal pathology through the optical system and the ultrasound transducer (Fig. 1.3). The ultrasound scanning plane of the instrument is directed to a 12 o'clock position, whereas the connecting cable of the endoscope is in the 6 o'clock position. The length of the insertion tube measures 125 cm, thereby allowing the placement of the ultrasound probe into the third part of the duodenum. The transducer is designed with 10 mm radius and generates a 100° real-time sector scan of high resolution.

The latest developments in curved linear array ultrasound endoscopes are incorporated in the Pentax-Hitachi FG 34 UX and FG 38 UX (Fig 1.4). These ultrasound gastroscopes are oblique, forward viewing endoscopes with an ultrasound transducer mounted on the tip of the instrument.

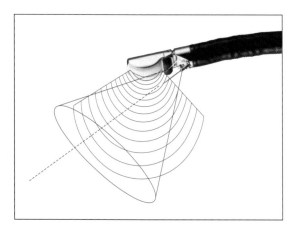

Fig. 1.3

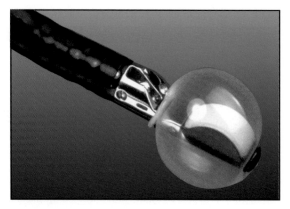

Fig. 1.5

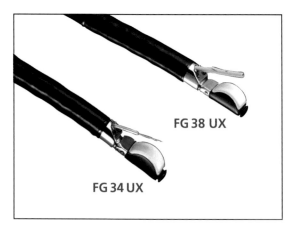

FG 38 UX

FG 34 UX

Fig. 1.4

The distal rigid portion of the gastroscope provides a 60° oblique forward view. The instrument channel outlet guides endoscopic accessories into the same direction. The electronic curved array transducer generates a 120° sector scan in the longitudinal plane, with the scanning direction along the axis of the gastroscope. The optical axis and the working channel are in the same plane, thus allowing visualization of interventional instrumentation in the endoscopic as well as in the ultrasound image. This facilitates EUS guided procedures such as Fine-Needle Aspiration biopsy (FNA), Fine-Needle Injection (FNI), or single-step placement of stents for drainage of pancreatic pseudocysts.

The transducer frequency can be selected from between 5 to 10 MHz, depending on the Ultrasound Base Unit, in order to optimize axial resolution and penetration depth according to the clinical require-

ments. A water-filled balloon (Fig 1.5) may be attached to the transducer to improve acoustic coupling and to optimize visualization of the region of interest. The balloon is secured by a double attachment. Filling and emtying of the balloon is controlled by the air/water and suction valves of the endoscope. For direct water instillation into the stomach, approximately 200 to 300 ccm water should be delivered through the working channel, e.g. by an automatic water supply source.

The major difference between the above mentioned models are working channels of 2.0 and 3.2 mm diameter (Table 1.1). This results in different outer diameters of the insertion tube. All other features and control functions of the endoscope are identical to those of conventional fiberoptic endoscopes. Tip deflection and precise positioning of the transducer can be accomplished with the control knobs. Air/water and suction valves at the control body facilitate insufflation and suction.

Endoscopic visualization is performed by connecting the umbilical cable of the endoscope to a conventional Halogen or Xenon light source which also supplies air and water.

Specifications of longitudinal ultrasound gastroscopes manufactured by Olympus are listed in Table 1.2. Other companies (e.g. Toshiba) have recently joined this area, but experience with their instruments is limited.

Current developments in system design for Endoscopic Ultrasound (EUS) favor the combination of an Universal Ultrasound System (Fig1.6) with probes for radial and longitudinal scanning. This concept is highly economical as the Ultrasound System can be used for general ultrasound applications

Table 1.1. Specifications of PENTAX/HITACHI Echoendoscopes

	FG-34UX	FG-36UX	FG-38UX
Optical system	fiberoptic	fiberoptic	fiberoptic
Direction of view	60° forward oblique	60° forward oblique	60° forward oblique
Field of view	105°	105°	105°
Tip deflection U/D	130/130°	130/130°	130/130°
Tip deflection R/L	120/120°	120/120°	120/120°
Rigid distal OD probe (mm)	12.0 × 12.8	12.0 × 12.8	12.0 × 12.8
Rigid distal OD optics (mm)	12.5	13.0	13.5
Insertion tube OD (mm)	11.5	12.1	12.8
Instrument channel ID (mm)	2.0	2.4	3.2
Working length (mm)	1250	1250	1250
Total length (mm)	1600	1600	1600
Elevator mechanismen	no	yes	no
US frequencies (MHz)	4.5 – 10.0	4.5 – 10.0	4.5 – 10.0
US scanning angle	120° longitud.	120° longitud.	120° longitud.
US scanning system	Convex 10R	Convex 10R	Convex 10R
Acoustic coupling	balloon	balloon	balloon
US display modes	B/CFM/CFA	B/CFM/CFA	B/CFM/CFA
US processor	HITACHI	HITACHI	HITACHI
	EG-3630U	**EG 3630UR**	**FG 3630UR**
Optical system	video	video	fiberoptic
Direction of view	60° forward oblique	forward	forward
Field of view	130°	120°	105°
Tip deflection U/D	130/130°	130/130°	130/130°
Tip deflection R/L	120/120°	120/120°	120/120°
Rigid distal OD probe (mm)	12.0 × 12.8	12.6	12.6
Rigid distal OD optics (mm)	13.0	12.0	12.0
Insertion tube OD (mm)	12.1	12.1	12.1
Instrument channel ID (mm)	2.4	2.4	2.4
Working length (mm)	1250	1250	1250
Total length (mm)	1575	1575	1575
Elevator mechanismen	yes	no	no
US frequencies (MHz)	4.5 – 10.0	4.5 – 10.0	4.5 – 10.0
US scanning angle	120° longitud.	270° radial	270° radial
US scanning system	Convex 10R	Convex 6R	Convex 6R
Acoustic coupling	balloon	balloon	balloon
US display modes	B/CFM/CFA	B/CFM/CFA	B/CFM/CFA
US processor	HITACHI	HITACHI	HITACHI

Table 1.2. Specifications of Olympus Echoendoscopes

Company		Olympus	Olympus	Olympus
Model Name		GF-UMD 140P	GF-UCT 140-AL5	GF-UC 140P-AL5
Endoscopic Functions				
Optical System	Field of View	100°	100°	100°
	Direction of View	55° Forward Oblique	55° Forward Oblique	55° Forward Oblique
	Depth of Field	3 ~ 100 mm	3 ~ 100 mm	3 ~ 100 mm
Insertion Tube	Distal End OD	14.4 mm	14.6 mm	14.2 mm
	Flexible Tube OD	11.8 mm	12.6 mm	11.8 mm
	Working Length	1244 mm	1250 mm	1250 mm
Instrument Channel	Channel Inner Diameter	2.8 mm	3.7 mm	2.8 mm
	Min. Visible Distance	6 mm	6 mm	6 mm
	Forceps Elevator		yes	yes
Bending Section	Angulation Range	UP 130°, DOWN 90° RIGHT 90° LEFT 90°	UP 130° DOWN 90° RIGHT 90° LEFT 90°	UP 130° DOWN 90° RIGHT 90°, LEFT 90°
Total Length		1624 mm	1575 mm	1575 mm
Ultrasonic Functions				
Display Mode		B-mode	B-mode, M-mode, D-mode, Flow-mode, Powerflow-mode	B-mode, M-mode, D-mode, Flow-mode, Powerflow-mode
Scanning Method		Mechanical sector scanning	Electrical curved linear array	Electrical curved linear array
Scanning Direction		Parallel to the insertion direction	Parallel to the insertion direction	Parallel to the insertion direction
Frequency		7,5 MHz	5, 6, 7.5, 10 MHz	5, 6, 7.5, 10 MHz
Scanning Range		270°	180°	180°
Contacting Method		Balloon Method, Sterile De-aerated Water Immersion Method	Balloon Method, Sterile De-aerated Water Immersion Method	Balloon Method, Sterile De-aerated Water Immersion Method
Compatible Processors		EU-M30, EU-M20 Olympus	SSD-5500PHD, SSD-5000PHD Aloka	SSD-5500PHD, SSD-5000PHD Aloka

when it is not used for EUS applications. A family of Ultrasound Base Systems is available, covering the entire performance range including compact black and white units and fully digital high end systems.

The recent introduction of fully digital ultrasound systems represents a milestone in the development of this imaging modality and will also expand the diagnostic capabilities of Endoscopic Ultrasound (EUS) due to further improvements in image quality.

Digital ultrasound systems are PC based and operate under standard software like Windows NT as the user interface.

The core of such an advanced ultrasound system is the Digital Beamformer (Fig 1.7), which is a highly specialized, rapid, and flexible computer designed for ultrasound functionality. The Digital Beamformer controls all acoustic parameters in real-time, a major technological breaktrough. In comparison to conventional analog beamformers, it performs all functions an order of magnitude faster, with more precision and reproducibility. The incorporated F1-Imaging technique generates a narrow beam profile by multiple apodization (frequency, amplitude, wave form) of the emitting signals, steering the different transducer elements and expanding the focus

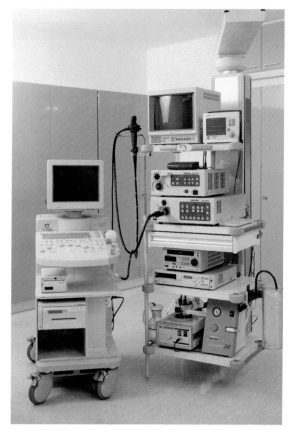

Fig. 1.6

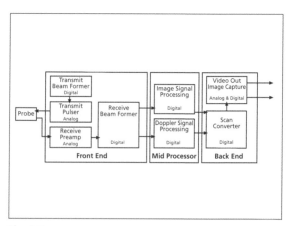

Fig. 1.7

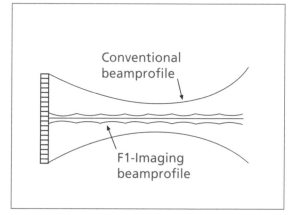

Fig. 1.8

range from the near field distally to the far field (Fig. 1.8). The result is better contrast and improved spatial and lateral resolution over the entire depth of the image.

In combination with the innovative Multi-Layer Transducer Technology, the frequency bandwidth of transducers can be increased between 4.5 MHz – 10 MHz allowing for multiple frequencies with the same instrument. This feature results in better visualization of deeper regions by selection of a lower frequency and improved resolution of wall structures by choosing a higher frequency.

Digital image processing algorithm facilitate speckle reduction in real-time, resulting in better homogeneity and reduced noise. Digital filtering algorithms can also increase Doppler sensitivity and reduce motion artifacts, thereby simplifying visualization of blood flow in EUS applications.

Finally, PC-based digital ultrasound systems offer efficient image management and networking capabilities.

J. Janssen · L. Greiner

CHAPTER 2
Indications

Endoscopic ultrasound is usually performed at the end of the diagnostic workup in order to answer one or more specific questions. Therefore, it is useful to be fully aware of the indications that are currently established (Table 2.1), those which are under investigation (Table 2.2), and those which are now obsolete (Table 2.3).

The capability of visualizing wall layers with a high resolution qualifies EUS as the method of choice to other imaging modalities such as CT or MR in imaging luminal lesions. Esophageal and rectal cancer are treated differently in multimodal therapeutic protocols, depending on the local stage of the carcinoma prior to treatment. There are some preliminary data suggesting that neoadjuvant protocols may also be useful in locally advanced gastric cancer. Whereas EUS nodal staging of esophageal carcinoma is relatively reliable, this does not apply to gastric cancer. It is difficult to correctly count all enlarged paragastric lymph nodes, since endosonographic imaging of the paragastric space is normally achieved by multiple, partly-overlapping scans.

In analogy to carcinomas, the *staging of gastrointestinal lymphomas*, lymphomas of the mucosa-associated lymphatic tissue (MALT) or systemic lymphomas with secondary infiltration of the stomach, can best be done by EUS. Therapy depends on the histological classification into high grade and low grade lymphomas and, especially in the latter case, on the local extent or multifocal infiltration of the tumor.

Small *pancreatic tumors* can be better visualized by EUS than by all other currently available imaging modalities. Therefore, EUS is a suitable diagnostic tool for the localization of small neuroendocrine tumors that have been previously diagnosed clinically by the presence of endocrine symptoms. The detection of duodenal neuroendocrine tumors is less effective. In the case of pancreatic carcinoma, pretreatment imaging is used primarily to decide on the local operability of the tumor. This includes detection of invasion of the mesenteric or celiac artery

Table 2.1. Generally accepted indications for EUS of the upper gastrointestinal tract

Staging of esophageal cancer
Staging of gastric cancer
Staging of malignant gastric lymphoma
Assessing operability of pancreatic cancer
Localisation of pancreatic neuroendocrine tumors
Staging of cancer of the papilla of Vater
Staging of ductal biliary cancer
Submucosal tumors, extramural impressions
Exclusion of pseudoachalasia
Giant gastric folds
Intramural gastric varices
EUS guided FNA of paraesophageal tumors
EUS guided FNA of pancreatic lesions
EUS guided FNA of the left adrenal gland
EUS guided FNA of intramural tumors (suspected metastatic intramural disease)

Table 2.2. Indications for EUS of the upper gastrointestinal tract under discussion

Achalasia
Follow- up after surgery of esophageal or gastric cancer
Follow- up after radiation and/or chemotherapy for esophageal cancer
Esophageal varices (treatment success)
Staging of lung cancer
Mediastinal staging of malignant lymphoma
Chronic pancreatitis
Detection of biliary stones
EUS guided FNA of submucosal tumors
EUS guided drainage of pancreatic pseudocysts

and its branches, the portal venous system, or neighboring organs. Although small carcinomas of about 1 cm in diameter can be visualized by EUS, early detection of small but asymptomatic tumors is rarely

Table 2.3. Questionable indications/contraindications for EUS of the upper gastrointestinal tract

Lack of consequence of the EUS result (known M1 stage, bad performance status of the patient (or inoperability)

Indeterminate or benign gastric or esophageal ulcers

Early detection of Barrett's adenocarcinoma

successful, as EUS is not a suitable screening method. Periampullary carcinomas and tumors of the papilla of Vater normally cause jaundice in the early stages of the disease, thereby usually resulting in prompt diagnostic imaging which often allows treatment in curative intent. EUS can successfully be used for the staging of malignancies of the papilla of Vater, but it cannot adequately differentiate adenomas from early stage carcinomas.

EUS is suitable to identify *submucosal tumors*, to define their layer of origin in the wall, and to describe criteria that help to differentiate between high and low risk lesions. Histopathologically accurate results, however, cannot be expected. Extramural impressions on the wall, as part of the differential diagnosis of submucosal tumors, can also be detected reliably.

Further indications for EUS are *giant gastric folds* and suspected *fundal varices* which are better classified by EUS than conventional endoscopy. The significance of endosonographic examination of esophageal varices or detection of perforating veins feeding subepithelial varices and the risk of recurrent bleeding have yet to be evaluated in further studies.

The role of EUS in the *follow- up during or after tumor therapy* (surgical, medical or radiological) has not yet been well defined. In the case of radiotherapy and/or chemotherapy, EUS cannot adequately differentiate between residual tumor and fibrous or inflammatory tissue reaction. It seems that EUS is highly sensitive in detecting lymph node or anastomotic tumor recurrences, but there is a considerable lack of specificity which makes the use of EUS in this setting debatable.

EUS is always problematic in *mucosal lesions* suspicious of malignancy, but not histologically confirmed. EUS is not able to differentiate between hypoechoic inflammatory and tumorous wall infiltration. Therefore, it is of no use to examine histologically benign ulcers or patients with severe esophagitis. For early detection of Barrett's related adenocarcinoma, mapping biopsies are much more useful than EUS. Inflammatory processes may even

infiltrate into the adventitia of the esophagus or beyond the gastric serosa mimicking stage T3 malignant disease.

Achalasia may show thickening of the circular layer of the muscularis propria, but it is primarily diagnosed clinically (endoscopically/radiologically) and proven by manometry. EUS is probably able to reveal so called pseudoachalasia due to intra- or extramural tumors.

The role of EUS in *biliary diseases* is not quite clear. EUS can detect small calculi within the common bile duct or gall bladder, but there are other highly sensitive and specific methods such as transcutaneous ultrasound and ERCP, or, more recently, MRCP. EUS may be indicated in borderline situations to identify microlithiasis without having the patient subjected to the risks of more invasive ERCP. Ductal biliary neoplasms can be staged by EUS. In some cases, intraductal ultrasound may be preferable.

Parenchymal and ductal abnormalities or stone formation in chronic pancreatitis can easily be visualized by EUS. Focal pancreatitis may result in images comparable to pancreatic carcinoma. The classification of hypoechoic areas in chronic pancreatitis remains problematic. EUS guided FNA is helpful when tumorous tissue can be aspirated. EUS, with or without FNA, might elucidate the reason for incomplete filling of the pancreatic duct on ERCP. Recent reports show good results of EUS guided internal drainage of pancreatic pseudocysts (see Part 5).

Staging of *bronchial carcinoma* can in part be done by EUS since it gives an insight into the dorsal paraesophageal mediastinum. In this context, EUS guided fine- needle aspiration biopsy is useful in certain cases to obtain the primary histology or to prove nodal metastasis in contralateral or subcarinal lymph nodes. Biopsy of paraesophageal lesions may also be useful in other situations involving a suspected malignancy.

Further indications for *EUS-FNA* are pathological findings in the left adrenal gland, pancreas, the paragastric lesions, and occasionally intramural tumors (see Part 4). Intramural metastatic disease resulting from carcinoma can be proven, whereas the differentiation between high risk and low risk stromal tumors is often not possible due the small specimen obtained by EUS guided fine-needle aspiration biopsy.

There are hardly any contraindications to EUS. The patient has to give informed consent and should be cooperative, which can usually be achieved by adequate sedation. Of course, EUS should only be done when therapeutic consequences are expected.

CHAPTER 3

Examination Technique and General Principles

J. Janssen · L. Greiner

Introduction

The principle of endoscopically introducing an ultrasound scanner into the gastrointestinal tract allows high frequency ultrasound to be used for the exploration of mural gastrointestinal processes as well as extramural structures in close proximity to the lumen. This results in images of high resolution which are superior to those obtained with all other imaging modalities currently used in clinical practice. Standard echoendoscopes work at frequencies between 7.5 and 12 MHz, thereby generating a point to point resolution of less than 2 mm. The penetration depth is limited to 3 to 5 cm, as high frequency scanners have the disadvantage of increased energy absorption by the scanned tissue compared to low frequency scanners.

These technical limitations and the variable anatomy of the gastrointestinal tract, which restricts the possible transducer positions, are the main reasons why endoscopic ultrasound (EUS) cannot be used as a screening method like transcutaneous ultrasound, which allows a complete overview of all organs of the abdomen. EUS is mostly used for well-defined indications when the high resolution of this method is required. Thus, EUS is often the final imaging procedure in the diagnostic process.

Gastrointestinal lesions should always be inspected first with a standard endoscope by the endosonographer himself, because the forward optical system allows a better macroscopic evaluation of the size and topography of the lesion than the side-viewing optics of the echoendoscope. Subsequent EUS does then not require endoscopic visualization in most cases. Furthermore, in the case of stenosis, standard endoscopy provides information on the perforation risk with the thicker echoendoscope.

Table 3.1. Tasks before EUS examination

Rechecking of the indication
Reviewing all available diagnostic imaging studies (e.g. CT-scans and transcutaneous ultrasound)
Endoscopy of mural lesions
Confirmation of blood coagulation status before EUS guided FNA biopsy
Written informed consent by the patient

Before performing endoscopic ultrasound, all diagnostic results, especially CT-scans, should be reviewed and available (Table 3.1). In abdominal lesions, such as in the pancreas, a transcutaneous ultrasound by the endosonographer himself is recommend, since it may give a better overall understanding of the topographic relations of pathological findings than endoscopic ultrasound. This makes the interpretation of EUS images easier and more reliable.

Preparation of the Patient

The patient provides written informed consent prior to the examination, as is requested for other invasive procedures. In comparison to standard upper gastrointestinal endoscopy, the risks are similar except for the increased danger of aspiration due to the instillation of water into the stomach during the examination.

When planning an EUS guided needle puncture, the patient has to be adequately informed as well. In the diagnostic setting, a fine needle is generally used which rarely causes complications such as perforation of intestinal organs or bleeding. In theory, metastatic seeding within the puncture channel or infections are possible adverse effects and must be discussed with the patient. In the literature, complications are rare and are mainly described after puncture of cystic pancreatic lesions. A platelet count over 80 000 and a prothrombin time with an INR<1,5 are sufficient to perform fine needle aspiration biopsy. In cases of more severely impaired clotting parameters, an individual decision has to be made balancing the potential benefit from the puncture against the risk of the procedure.

Dilation of a stenosis is sometimes necessary before endosonography and constitutes the highest risk of this examination. Therefore, the necessity of this maneuver should be carefully considered. In some cases, the advanced stage of a malignant disease is evident from other findings (e.g. CT-scan). EUS is thus not really necessary, as the indication for a palliative treatment regimen is already established. In other cases, EUS with a miniprobe can render dilation unnecessary and solve the diagnostic problem.

EUS is usually performed with a mild sedation, e.g. with intravenous midazolam, and continuous monitoring of the pulse, blood pressure, and oxygenation. After the procedure, the patient must be kept under adequate surveillance until the sedation has worn off.

The examination always starts with the patient lying on his left side. In most cases, there is no need for changing the position during the procedure. Occasionally, it is easier to scan the pancreatic head or the ampulla of Vater with the patient in a prone position. Therefore, positioning the patient on his left side with his left arm behind his body, as routinely done for ERCP examinations, may be recommended to facilitate repositioning into a prone position during the examination.

It is sometimes useful to inhibit peristalsis during the examination with butylscopolamine or glucagon in order to prevent the stomach from emptying too quickly after filling it with water. In this case, the patient may also need to be turned onto his right side to better visualize antral mural findings after water filling.

Tissue Contact of the Transducer

Gas between the transducer and the gastrointestinal surface prevents the generation of satisfactory images of mural processes and the surrounding extramural structures. The transducer can be tightly pressed against the wall, thus removing the gas barrier and allowing direct contact. This technique can be effective in examining structures outside of the gastrointestinal wall. If the wall itself is the region of interest, strong pressure must be avoided (Fig. 3.1), as it causes fusion of neighboring wall layers in the ultrasound image. This makes detailed differentiation of the layers impossible, which is essential for reliable staging of intramural carcinomas.

Filling the stomach with water provides an excellent scanning field without creating any pressure on the wall and is advantageous whenever possible (Fig. 3.2). In the esophagus, the use of water cannot generally be recommended due to the increased risk of aspiration. In the duodenum, water often disappears quickly, despite inhibition of peristalsis

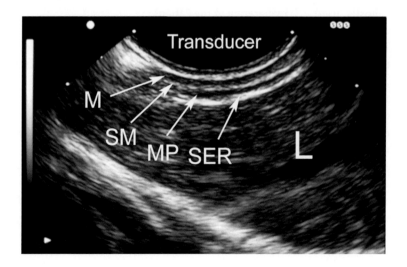

Fig. 3.1. Optimal transducer contact. The transducer has close contact to the gastric wall of the lesser curvature. The wall layers are even and can be well differentiated, indicating the application of minimal pressure. *M,* Mucosa; *SM,* submucosa; *MP,* muscularis propria; *SER,* serosa; *L,* left liver lobe

Fig. 3.2. Transducer contact. Water filling of the gastrointestinal organs provides optimal conditions to examine the wall without compressing the wall layers. Therefore, this technique should be used whenever possible. In the esophagus, it should generally be avoided due to the enhanced risk of aspiration

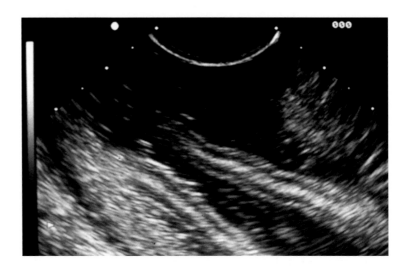

Fig. 3.3. Transducer contact. In this case, the close contact between transducer and gastric wall is achieved by means of the water-filled balloon. This gastric carcinoma (*TU*) is characterized by a hypoechoic transmural tumor infiltration and local penetration of the serosa (*arrow*, T3 carcinoma). Such findings can correctly be staged even when exerting major pressure onto the wall. *B*, Balloon; *MP*, muscularis propria

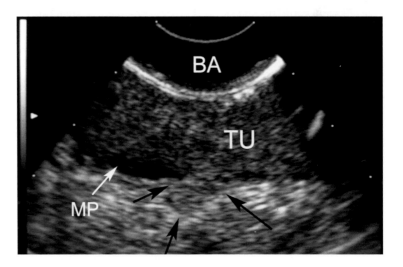

with butylscopolamine or glucagon. For these anatomical regions, the transducer should be covered with a balloon, which is then filled with water to enable sufficient contact to the wall without producing too much pressure (Fig. 3.3). Furthermore, intraluminal air should be removed by suction to improve contact.

EUS Orientation and Examination Strategies

The echoendoscope is equipped with a side-viewing optical system, which allows endoscopic orientation. Endoscopic visualization is necessary for the exam-

ination of small mural lesions, to facilitate the passage through the pylorus, and occasionally to allow faster access to the ampulla of Vater. However, careful inspection of mural processes with a forward viewing optical system cannot be replaced by this side-viewing technique.

EUS of larger mural lesions and extramural structures can be performed under ultrasonographic visualization only, without the help of endoscopic orientation. Orientation is established in analogy to transcutaneous ultrasound by anatomic landmarks, i.e. larger vessels (aorta, splenic and portal vein, inferior vena cava) and the pancreas.

Endosonography allows the visualization of the aorta from its origin at the aortic valve down into the abdomen just beyond the origin of the superior mesenteric artery. The ascending thoracic aorta has a small ultrasonographic gap caused by interference of air located in the trachea, which is situated partially posterior to the aortic arch. As the topographic relationship between the aorta and the organs in the mediastinum and middle abdomen is usually reproducible, it is helpful to localize the aorta whenever the orientation is lost.

While the aorta represents the longitudinal landmark in the mediastinum and upper abdomen, the pancreas can be used as cross-sectional landmark in the abdomen. The pancreatic head has a close relationship to the inferior vena cava, to the right kidney, and to the adrenal gland, whereas the body and the tail are in close proximity to the left adrenal gland, the left kidney, and the spleen.

Using these landmarks one may find the spleen in the following way:

1. Coming from the mediastinum the descending thoracic aorta is followed through the diaphragmatic hiatus into the abdomen.
2. Ventrally to the origin of the superior mesenteric artery, the pancreatic body is visualized in a longitudinal section.
3. Rotating the echoendoscope to the right shifts the scanning area to the left side of the aorta towards the pancreatic tail, allowing the visualization of the left adrenal gland between the pancreatic body and the psoas muscle.
4. Further rotation to the right and cautious retraction reveals the pancreatic tail, which ends in the splenic hilum.

Similar algorithms can be drawn up for all structures of the dorsal mediastinum and the upper half of the abdomen.

It is important to be aware that transducer rotation will lead to visualization of structures in the direction of the rotation, if the transducer starts in a ventral position. Rotation will show contralateral structures relative to the direction of rotation, if the transducer is orientated dorsally when the rotation is initiated.

To scan the complete circumference of the esophagus, the stomach and the duodenum, it is necessary to repeatedly perform 360° rotations while the transducer is withdrawn in a stepwise fashion. This maneuver can only be successfully carried out if circular contact to the wall is established (see above). Whereas complete examination of the esophagus can usually be achieved, it is often difficult to completely visualize the stomach and the duodenum. In particular, the fundus, the antrum, and the angularis area remain problematic zones, because these locations necessitate contorted scope positions. In these cases rotation of the transducer simultaneously induces movements of the echoendoscope in the longitudinal axis, making it difficult to ensure complete inspection of the gastric wall. The same problem occurs when trying to localize paragastric lymph nodes.

There are several methods of performing EUS in a systematic fashion. Many examiners prefer to introduce the instrument deeply into the duodenum and to inspect the luminal wall and surrounding structures by rotating and retracting the transducer in a step by step fashion. On the other hand, it has also been proven effective to first examine the paraesophageal mediastinum followed by the middle and left abdomen after introducing the probe. The advantage of this technique is that there is no need to inflate air into the stomach thus improving the examination conditions. Furthermore, there are several indications for EUS, such as the staging of esophageal cancer, where the passage of the transducer through the pylorus is not required. Shortening the duration of the examination without loss of diagnostic information is desirable for the patient's comfort, and this should be done whenever possible.

As EUS is not a screening method, but is only performed for certain, specific indications, the examiner always has to be aware of which regions are to be explored in a given case. This is especially true for lymph node staging in gastrointestinal cancer, e. g. for the celiac region in esophageal cancer.

Image Orientation on the Monitor

There is no established convention yet concerning image orientation on the monitor. In analogy to transcutaneous ultrasound, it seems logical to present oral ("cranial") structures on the left and pedal ("caudal") structures on the right side of the monitor. This image orientation is therefore used in this book.

Of course, this orientation may generate images which are contradictory to those of transcutaneous ultrasound. For example when retracting the dorsal-

Fig. 3.4. Image inversion. Scanning from the posterior wall of the duodenal bulb shows the pancreatic head and body, including the characteristic surrounding vessels. The image orientation (*right/left*) is inverted compared with the transcutaneous ultrasound technique. *P*, Pancreas; *CON*, confluence; *SV*, splenic vein; *SMA*, superior mesenteric artery

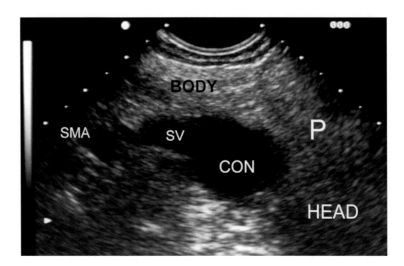

ly turned probe through the duodenal bulb, the pancreatic head shows up at the right side of the body and the confluence of the splenic and superior mesenteric vein is visualized at the right side of the superior mesenteric artery (Fig. 3.4). Nevertheless this orientation should be maintained in order to guarantee the interobserver comparability of EUS images.

Endoscopic Color Flow and Conventional Doppler Ultrasonography

The electronic convex transducer enables blood flow visualization by pulsed doppler, color flow and power mode technique. The theoretical background and further details of these techniques are not presented in this book. Special literature on this subject is available.

No studies have yet been published which prove the necessity of conventional Doppler and color flow doppler in endoscopic ultrasonography. Nevertheless, there is no doubt among most users that color flow Doppler improves visualization by quickly allowing the endosonographer to distinguish between arteries, veins and other tubular anechoic structures. Endosonographic puncture of an anechoic lesion, such as within the pancreas, should only be done after exclusion of perfusion of the lesion by Doppler, because puncture of an arterial aneurysm may proof to be detrimental.

In some cases it is helpful to use color flow EUS to look for fundic varices. Pilot studies show that EUS is more sensitive and specific than endoscopy for this purpose. The color flow imaging of perforating veins that feed subepithelial esophageal varices and visualization of sclerotherapy or banding effects can easily be done with the convex scanner, but the clinical value of this indication for EUS has not yet been clearly defined.

Documentation

As EUS is a real-time method, it is favorable to record representative sequences of each examination on video tapes. Prints and photographs can only demonstrate characteristic sections of a finding, whereas the video shows the complete process and its relation to the surrounding organs and vessels. Thus, this medium has proven to be especially suitable for conferences and discussions with colleagues from other (e.g. surgical) departments. Furthermore, the video allows critical evaluation of the EUS examination, which is important in cases of discrepancies with other diagnostic or postoperative findings.

Terminology

Image description in EUS follows the terminology guidelines used in transcutaneous ultrasound. The brightness represents the echogenity of a structure and is described by the terms anechoic for black, hypoechoic or hyporeflective for dark, and hyperechoic or hyper-reflective for bright structures. The terms "density" and "intensity" are restricted to CT and MR imaging.

The examiner should always analyze the homogeneity of a process, the characteristics of its outer border (smooth, rough, dentated etc.), and its size measured in at least two dimensions. Findings in the esophagus should further be characterised by the insertion depth of the echoendoscope. For comparison with other imaging modalities and for surgical planning, it is important to describe the relationship of the lesion to the neighboring vessels and other important structures. The description should not contain any diagnoses, as these should be separately summarized at the end of the report.

For tumor staging the appropriate classification is applied. The most important classifications for upper gastrointestinal EUS are listed in short form in the appendix of this book. TNM stages derived from EUS are characterised by the prefix "u" in differentiation to other staging modalities (e. g. prefix "p" for pathological and "c" for clinical staging).

Pitfalls and Artifacts

Problems in EUS may arise due to physical artifacts and certain typical pitfalls (Table 3.2). Sometimes however, artifacts are characteristic diagnostic criteria, as e.g. the acoustic shadowing in stone disease. A knowledge of these pitfalls and artifacts is essential, as they can often be overcome by optimizing the examination technique.

In order to evaluate the thickness of the gastrointestinal wall correctly, it is mandatory to position the transducer at a right angle to the wall. Oblique position of the transducer will result in an overestimation of the thickness of the wall layers or a mural tumor (Fig. 3.5). The correct transducer position is difficult to establish especially in certain regions of the stomach such as the fundus and the angularis. In these cases, inversion and torsion of the echoendoscope is required. Sometimes, it is helpful to change the patient's position.

When a tumor stenosis cannot be traversed by the echoendoscope, there is also the risk of overestimating the thickness of the process, because the tip of the echoendoscope will easily be bent towards the stenotic lumen. The image then shows more of the length, rather than the depth, of the tumor. Never-

Table 3.2. Pitfalls in EUS

Insufficient contact between the transducer and the gastrointestinal wall
Exertion of too much pressure onto the gastrointestinal wall
Tangential scanning of the gastrointestinal wall
Confusion of the scanning direction above a non-traversable tumor stenosis
Misinterpretation of hypoechoic inflammation as tumorous infiltration
Insufficient adjustment of the ultrasound system (gain, focus depth, sector size)
Misinterpretation of ultrasound artifacts

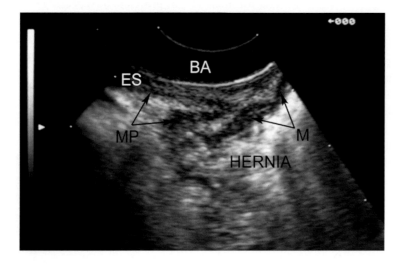

Fig. 3.5. Scanning angle. This example shows the transition of the distal esophagus (*ES*) into an axial hiatal hernia. The wall layers, especially the mucosa, show varying thicknesses of the same layer within the hernia, which results from tangential and rectangular scanning. *BA*, Balloon; *M*, mucosa; *MP*, muscularis propria

theless, tumor infiltration of neighboring structures can often be confirmed, even if the stenosis cannot be passed. In most cases, this finding demonstrates inoperability and indicates a palliative regimen, rendering dilation of the stenosis in order to perform a complete EUS examination unnecessary.

Pressure on the gastrointestinal wall by the transducer will prevent the exact differentiation of the wall layers. This may lead to an overstaging of T1-carcinomas, because the hypoechoic submucosal tumor infiltration cannot be distinguished from the muscularis propria. As already discussed, this problem may be overcome by minimizing pressure on the wall or reducing the amount of water in the balloon.

Some inflammatory reaction is found around most tumors. Since inflammatory infiltration produces the same hypoechoic pattern as tumor infiltration, this phenomenon may also result in an overstaging of T1 or T2 tumors. Sometimes, it is useful to move the transducer along the tumor and to observe whether the wall layers are immobile or slide against one another, thereby determining the infiltration depth.

Image quality always depends on the adjustment of the ultrasound system. The near and far gain must be adapted so that vessels appear anechoic but solid hypoechoic structures are still identifiable as such. There is no standard scanning position in EUS which allows a reproducible gain adjustment like in transcutaneous ultrasound where the standard scan through the right kidney and right liver lobe is used for this purpose. When adjusting the gain too high, solid tissue may be simulated within liquid structures, and when adjusting it too low, hypoechoic findings may appear as anechoic images. Therefore, permanent gain adjustment is necessary.

The focus or focus zone must correspond to the depth of the region of interest and should always be optimized in order to achieve the best lateral resolution in this area. Furthermore, the structures of interest should be positioned in the middle of the scanning sector, which should be kept narrow to improve lateral resolution.

The monitor image can be improved by adapting the image size and zooming into the region of interest. The point to point resolution is not affected by zooming, at least not with the usual EUS equipment.

Modern ultrasound machines reduce technical artifacts to a minimum. However, the same artifacts are to be expected in EUS as in transcutaneous ultrasound. The most important artifacts are listed below without going into a detailed explanation of their physical origin:

1. *Enhancement by transmission* occurs behind anechoic structures such as cysts. In these cases, the far gain has to be corrected.
2. A *shadow* (Fig. 3.6) is caused by strong reflecting agents such as gas/ air or structures which reflect and absorb ultrasound waves to a high degree (e.g. bones).
3. *Repetitive echoic bands* (Fig. 3.7) and the *mirror artifact* (Fig. 3.8) are caused by strong reflectors (e.g. ventilated lung) that lead to multiple reflections of the ultrasound beam. A special form of this situation is the reverberation artifact seen

Fig. 3.6. Artifacts: *shadow.* These large stones within a dilated pancreatic duct in the pancreatic head reveal a characteristic corresponding shadow (*SH*) due to complete ultrasound energy absorption and reflection. The small calculi (*arrows*) do not show this artifact.

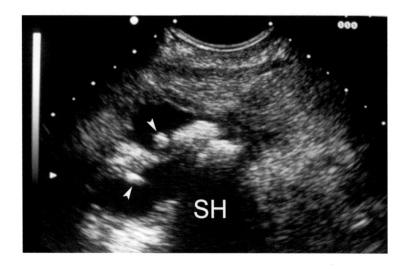

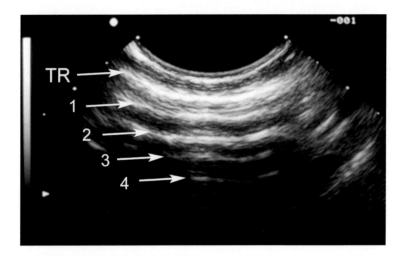

Fig. 3.7. Artifacts: *repetitive echoic bands*. The air filled trachea (*TR*) causes complete reflection of the ultrasound beams which return to the transducer at a preserved high energy level, thus causing re-reflection. The process occurs repeatedly. Four echoic bands (*arrow*) with decreasing brightness at equal intervals from the transducer appear on the monitor according to the time dependent representation of the reflections.

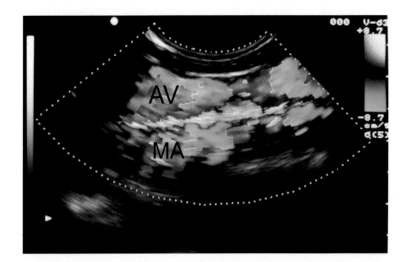

Fig. 3.8. Artifacts: *mirror artifact*. Strong reflectors such as the ventilated lung may cause a mirror artifact (*MA*). The virtual doubling of the azygos vein (*AV*) in B mode or color doppler ultrasound, as in this example, is quite frequent.

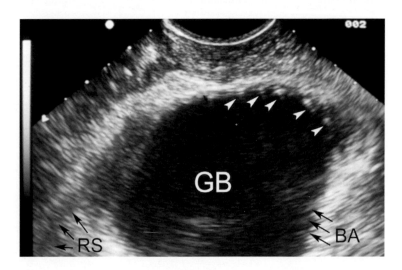

Fig. 3.9. Artifacts: *bow artifact, refractile shadow*, and "*comet's tail artifact*." The gallbladder (*GB*) normally has an anechoic bile filling. Strong reflectors in the near by surrounding tissue may lead to bow artifacts (*BA*). Ultrasound beams arriving tangentially at the gall bladder wall are not reflected in the same direction and cause the refractile shadow (*RS*). The cholesterol polyps of this gall bladder are characterized by discrete repetitive echoes (*arrowheads*), so-called "comet's tails," which also are typical of small gas pearls.

behind small air bubbles (*"comet's tail artifact"*, Fig. 3.9), which is characterized by narrow repetitive echoic bands at intervals equal to the bubble's size.

4. *Refractive shadows* (Fig. 3.9) are seen at the margins of rounded hypoechoic structures, such as cysts, because the echoes are refracted at these margins and do not return to the transducer.

5. *Bow artifacts* (Fig. 3.9) are caused by strong reflectors at the edge of anechoic areas if the focus has not been optimally adjusted. In this setting, bright bows appear within the anechoic zone, which correspond to the lateral resolution of the reflectors.

As gas is one of the most frequent causes of artifacts, it is evident that the balloon must always be carefully filled with water and air bubbles have to be eliminated.

Closing Remark

EUS, especially when using the longitudinal technique, requires a considerable amount training and technical skill before reliable and satisfactory results can be obtained. It is important to be aware of the normal anatomy. In addition, pathological findings should always be compared with other preoperative diagnostic imaging results and subsequently with postoperative findings, because only permanent feedback will help to improve EUS results. When beginning with EUS, one should not hesitate to discuss difficult cases with more experienced colleagues, as EUS results can decide the method of treatment, especially when multimodal therapeutic strategies are available, such as in esophageal cancer.

PART 2

Anatomy

(For abbreviations see page 175)

Normal Anatomy and Landmarks

U. Will · E. Burmester · J. Erk

Introduction

There has been international agreement on the orientation of images on the ultrasound screen. In longitudinal scans, cranial structures are shown on the left side and caudal structures on the right side. These guidelines have also been accepted for endosonography (EUS) in most parts of the world, with only a few exceptions. All anatomic findings shown here are demonstrated in the accepted manner. The left side of the endosonographic image indicates the cranial site, while the right side depicts the caudal site.

The curved array transducer produces a sector image parallel to the long axis of the endoscope. This may cause difficulties in ascertaining anatomic orientation, identifying structures, and interpreting findings. Therefore, it is important to know the anatomic landmarks that will enable the investigator to identify neighboring tissues, organs, and structures. Anatomically oriented endosonography is a key for the appropriate and successful use of longitudinal scanners.

To introduce anatomically standardized endosonographic images, some basic aspects are to be illustrated. If a straight and axially aligned endoscopic ultrasonographic transducer is directed ventrally, a rotation of the instrument to the right (clockwise) causes simultaneous rotation of the transducer to the right. The same principle applies with regard to rotations of the transducer to the left. In contrast, if the transducer is direted dorsally, rotation to the right generates an opposite shift of the scanning plane to the left because the transducer rotates to the left side.

After the guiding anatomic structures have been found (usually aorta or pancreas), the whole endoscope is rotated axialy to identify neighboring tissues and structures. If the orientation is lost, the instrument should be returned to its original posi-tion. A repeat attempt should be undertaken with a slightly angulated EUS tranducer, which is achieved by turning the big handle of the endoscope while simultaneously pushing the endoscope forward or withdrawing it.

Variation of the scanning planes is achieved by rotation of the endoscope with a straight or an angled transducer, i. e. an additional lateral angulation by manipulation of the small handle is rarely necessary. It is essential to imagine and understand the maneuvers described above, since there is no endoscopic image, only the endosonographic image to help with orientation.

It is advantageous to move the transducer along known guiding structures or landmarks, which facilitates orientation and allows anatomy-derived and systematic endosonographic examination. The endoscope should be rotated only slightly and all other manipulations such as angulation, advancement, or withdrawing should be performed slowly to avoid loss of orientation.

In certain cases, anatomic variations will necessiatate deviation from these suggested approaches. Clinicians should be quickly able to develop skills, which will allow them to perform appropriate endoscope manipulations. When evaluating the luminal masses of the upper gastrointestinal tract (esophagus, stomach, duodenum), dircet endoscopic visualization can be achieved to allow sufficient coupling of the transducer with the tissue of interest. This approach saves time, but carries the disadvantage that air insufflation is needed, which impairs the subsequent EUS examination.

The following chapters describe the EUS examination of guiding anatomic structures. The generation of EUS images is demonstrated, and then the stepwise process of proceeding from one guiding structure to another is presented. For a better orientation, several EUS pictures of the esophagus are marked on the enclosed computerized tomography (CT) scans. The positions of EUS transducer and endoscope in the stomach and duodenum are illustrated in some accompanying photographs and figures. These prints show an EUS transducer after dissection of the ventral part of the gastrointestinal tract during autopsy.

CHAPTER 4
Esophagus and Mediastinum: Imaging Techniques

U. Will · E. Burmester · J. Erk

(For abbreviations see page 175)

The wall layers of the upper gastrointestinal tract

1. Endoscopic visual control is only necessary for smaller mucosal and intramural lesions of the esophagus in order to facilitate positioning of the transducer. In these cases water-filling of the balloon is helpful.
2. After filling of the balloon, continuous suctioning of the esophageal lumen is helpful. Sometimes instillation of water into the esophagus is recommended, but it may be risky due to the danger of aspiration. Therefore if this is done, elevation of the head of the bed is recommended.
3. As the transducer is located distal to the endoscopic image, remember to withdraw the instrument slowly until the lesion is visible on the ultrasound image.
4. Remember the anatomy of the wall stuctures to define the depth of infiltrations.
5. Don't forget to image adjacent structures.

Mediastinum – Imaging Techniques

1. Introduce the instrument and advance it into the middle third of the esophagus.
2. Look for the mediastinal landmarks by rotating the instrument.

Note

If the transducer is *ventrally* directed, the scanning plane in the body moves in the direction of the rotation (right rotation moves the transducer to the right side of the body).

If the transducer is *dorsally* directed, the scanning plane moves in the opposite direction (right rotation moves the transducer to the left side of the body).

Your first landmark: the aorta, the azygos vein, and the spine

3. Rotate the axially directed instrument until you see the aorta as a broad vessel, which is usually scanned longitudinally and located dorsally and to the left.
4. Try to follow the vessel caudally by adapted rotation and stepwise advancement of the endoscope.

5. Rotate the instrument further to the left and reduce the pressure on the wall in order to see
   – the very small azygous vein,
   – the hyperechoic band of the spine.
6. Go back to the descending aorta and try to follow the vessel by adapted rotation and withdrawal until you reach the aortic arch.
7. After a slight angulation and rotation, you will see the left subclavian artery. Further rotation occasionally reveals the left common artery.
8. Further rotation and slow withdrawal of the instrument will lead you to the ascending aorta and the aortic valve.

Your second landmark: the pulmonary trunk

9. Turn the endoscope ventrally again and search for the aortic trunk.
10. By slightly rotating the tip of the transducer to the left the anechoic, typically round cross-sectional plane of the right pulmonary artery becomes visible.
11. Follow the vessel to its origin in the right ventricle.
12. You will see the left atrium close to your transducer.

Important, but difficult, third landmark: the trachea, the left and the right bronchus

13. Pull your instrument back when you see the right pulmonary artery.
14. You will only see parts of the trachea and the bronchial system due to the total reflection of the air near the right pulmonary artery.
15. The massive reverberation artifacts close to your transducer correspond to the trachea.
16. Use the trachea as a guiding structure and follow the bronchial system by rotating the instrument into the planes of the right bronchus and the left bronchus.

Your final landmark: the heart

17. By following your guiding structures, the pulmonary and the aortic trunks, you will reach the right and left atrium.
18. From to the cardia or with a cranial view from the gastric fundus: During rotation, you will see that the left ventricle consists of a thick muscle and that the right ventricle has a thinner wall.

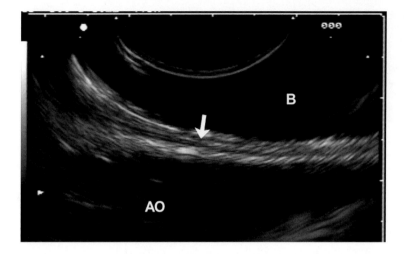

Fig. 4.1. Normal esophageal wall: The 7.5 MHz image demonstrates the normal EUS anatomy of the five layers ("arrow" – see legend Fig. 4.2) between the filled balloon and the aortic wall (arrow). The close contact with the aorta shows that the transducer is rotated to the descending part of the aorta and directed dorsally and to the left. The balloon is only partially filled with water in order to avoid artifacts form compression of the wall and to show all five layers. If the balloon is totally filled, the five layer structure will be reduced to three layers. Please also note the loss of normal stuctures in the upper and the lower third of the image due to the tangential scanning plane. You must move the instrument cranially or caudally for a better visualization. A systematic investigation of the whole wall is not required since EUS is indicated only for suspicious findings seen on standard endoscopy.

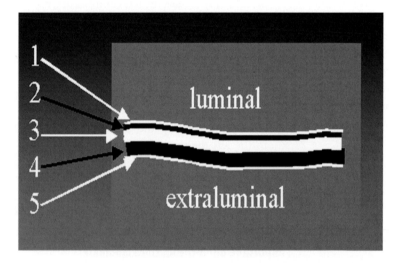

Fig. 4.2. Schematic image of the wall layers corresponding to 4.1.
1 interface echo
2 muscularis mucosae
3 submucosa
4 proper muscle layer
5 serosa

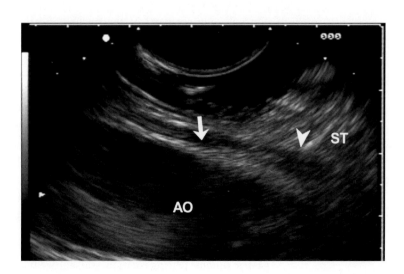

Fig. 4.3. Cardia: The EUS transducer is dorsally directed to depict the descending aorta (*AO*). In the lower third of the esophagus, a bandlike hypoechoic structure, the median side of the diaphragm (*arrow*), becomes visible. The cardia with a slight thickening of the muscular propria is now visible showing the lower esophageal sphincter. A careful angulation of the tip also allows a view of the fundic wall (*ST*).

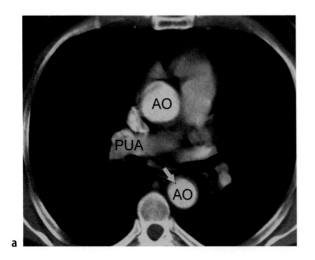

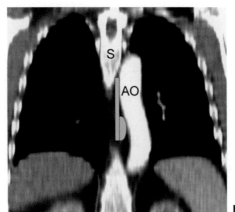

The first landmarks:
Descending aorta/azygos vein

Fig. 4.4 a–d. Descending aorta: After intubation of the esophagus, the endoscope is advanced into the middle part of the esophagus. Now the transducer should be rotated until a longitudinal section of the descending aorta is reached. This guiding structure can be followed caudally by pushing the instrument forward. The thoracic aorta, located dorsally in the mediastinum, is the main landmark for anatomically oriented EUS. Starting with the depiction of this anatomic structure, all observable organs can be imaged in a systematic manner in the mediastinum. **(a, b)** Simulations of the corresponding position of the ultrasound endoscope on various sections of a CT scan, **(c)** the proximal part of the descending aorta near the aortic arch, **(d)** the distal part of the descending aorta. The adjacent lung to the aorta generates reveberation echos (arrows in d).

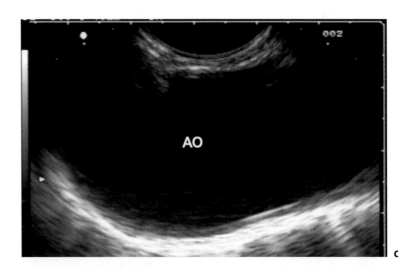

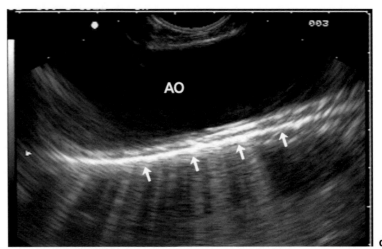

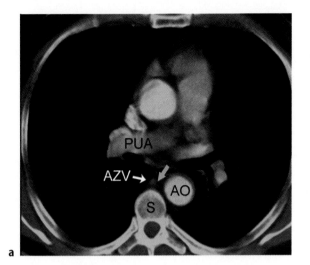

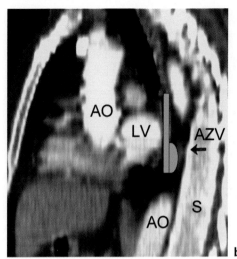

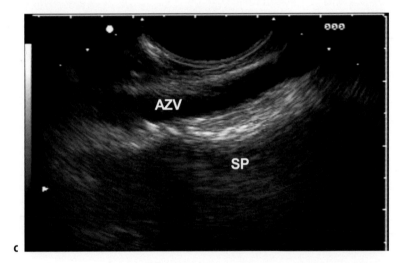

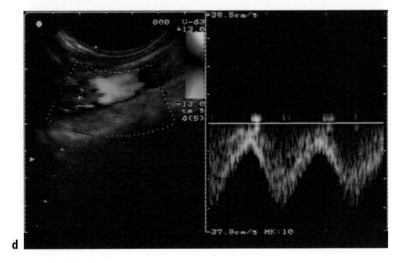

Fig. 4.5 (a–d) Azygos vein: Reducing the compression on the esophageal wall and rotating the endoscope further to the left the thin anechoic azygos vein, located to the right of the aorta and ventrally to the spine, will become visible. The spine will appear as a dense hyperechoic band with distal shadowing alternating with hypoechoic interruptions indicating the intervertebral discs. The color doppler mode **(d)** will easily identify the azygous vein if there is no compression on the vessel. **a, b** Simulations of the corresponding position of the echoendoscope on various sections of a CT scan.

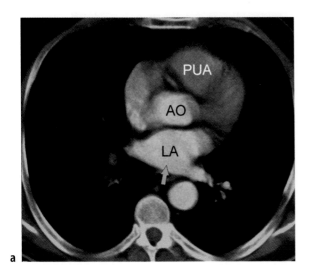

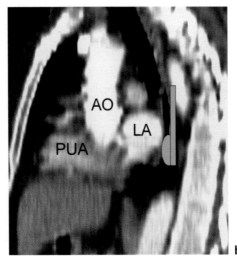

a   b

The second landmark:
Ascending aorta, aortic arch, pulmonary trunk

Fig. 4.6. Aortic arch and ascending aorta: Withdrawing the instrument slowly along the descending aorta, you will reach the proximal part of the aorta. Rotate the transducer into the aortic arch and advance into the ascending part. If the scanning plane is directed ventrally and slightly to the left, you will see the aortic valve, the left atrium dorsally between the aorta and the esophagus, and parts of the left ventricle with the mitral valve. The pulmonary artery is ventral to the aortic trunk. Pressing the transducer closer to the esophageal wall will produce better visualization of the aorta and its originating vessels. While the left subclavian artery can often be demonstrated, the left carotid artery and the brachiocephalic trunk can only infrequently be shown due to interposition of the lung. **a, b** Simulations of the corresponding position of the ultrasound endoscope on various sections of a CT scan.

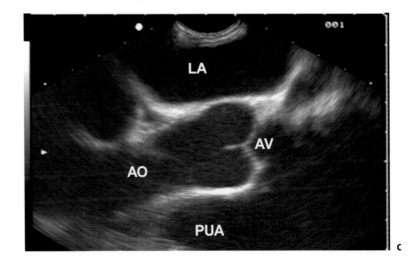

c

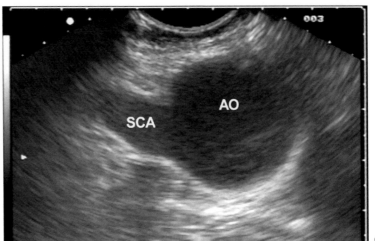

d

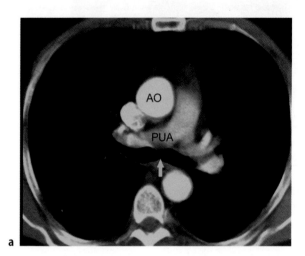

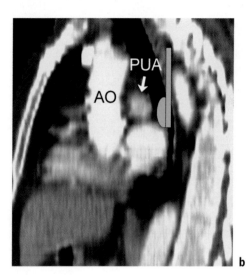

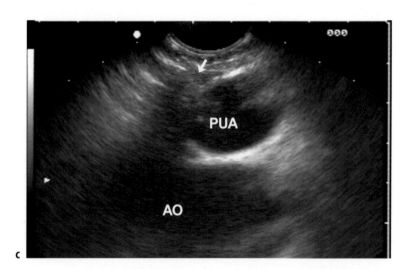

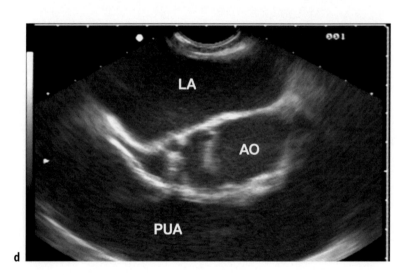

Fig. 4.7 a–d. Pulmonary trunk: By withdrawing the transducer from the ascending aorta, a round, anechoic orthograde view of the right pulmonary artery becomes clearly visible between the aorta and the esophageal wall. The reverberation artifacts cranially to the PUA mark the tracheal bifurcation (arrow in **c**). By rotating and slowly advancing the scope along the right pulmonary artery, the pulmonary trunk can be followed into the right ventricle. In the same ultrasound plane, the left atrium will appear as a large, anechoic lumen between the aorta and the transducer. **a, b** Simulations of the corresponding position of the ultrasound endoscope on various sections of a CT scan.

Third landmark: Trachea, Bronchus

Fig. 4.8. Trachea: Air produces a total reflection of the ultrasound waves. Therefore, EUS can only point out parts of the tracheal and bronchial system, demonstrated as hyperechoic echos from the cartilaginous wall and as reveberation echos in the air-filled lumen. Turn the instrument ventrally and search for the landmark of the right pulmonal artery (*PUA*), which is located just below the bifurcation, in order to find the trachea and the tracheal bifurcation. The massive reveberation echos of the trachea become visible by withdrawing the instrument in a longitudinal manner. Take care, not to mistake this structure with the spine, which is located dorsally and can produce a similar EUS-image.

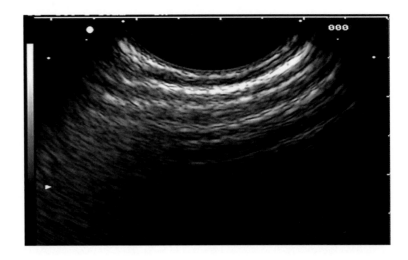

Fig. 4.9. Left main bronchus: Advance the instrument and suddenly the air- induced artifact that marks the tracheal bifurcation will disappear. Now follow the pearl-string like echoes along the main bronchus by slightly rotating the transducer to the left into the left main bronchus. Due to the smaller caliber of this structure, reduced air-artifacts allow a demonstration of the neighbouring structures, especially enlarged lymphnodes. The investigation of both peribronchial regions is important for the staging of bronchial carcinomas and both areas can be reached by EUS guided fine-needle puncture.

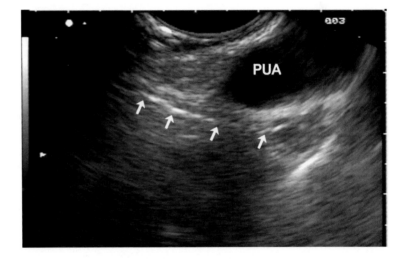

Fig. 4.10. Right main bronchus: The right main bronchus can be followed by going back to the tracheal bifurcation and rotating the transducer to the right. The imaging of the right bronchus requires a slight angulation of the EUS transducer in order to follow the typical wall-echoes of the bronchus, due to the greater distance from the esophagus. Adapation of the scanning plane by rotation of the instrument may be necssary.

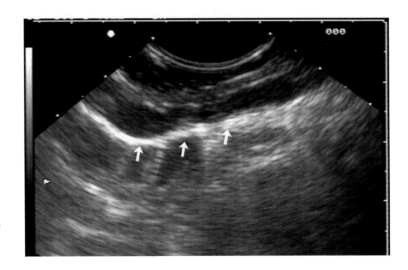

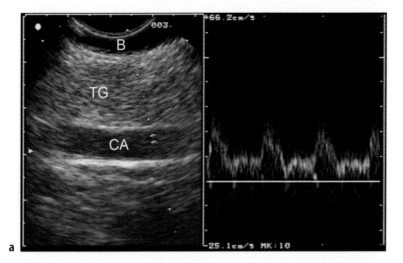

a

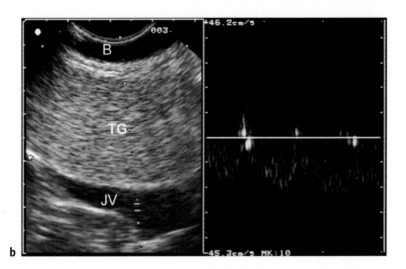

b

Fig. 4.11 a, b. Thyroid gland: You may pass the thyroid gland at the level of the upper esophageal spincter during the investigation of the proximal esophagus and trachea. While the left lobe of the gland is easy to visualize, scanning of the right lobe is often disturbed by reveberation artifacts due to the air-filled trachea. Up to now, there are no accepted indications for EUS-investigation of the thyroid gland, but there may be a clinical benefit in searching for small adenomas of the parathroid glands. The thyroid gland has a homogenous, intermediate echogenic pattern. Laterally, the neighboring vessels can be depicted and further differentiated by using the color Doppler or power Doppler mode. The thin esophageal wall is located between the filled balloon and the thyroid gland.

Fig. 4.12 a–c. Left atrium, right atrium: At the left atrium (*LA*), the pulmonary veins (*PUV*) and the left auricle can be imaged by slightly rotating the endoscope with simultaneous angulation. Using this ultrasound section plane, the mitral valve and the base of the left ventricle (*LV*) can be seen. By rotating to the right, the superior vena cava (*SCV*) and its entrance into the right atrium (*RA*) become visible behind the left atrium. Further rotation to the right or left with a slight angulation of the EUS transducer demonstrates the right and left ventricle, respectively. Investigation of the heart is important for staging advanced esophageal carcinomas that have the potential for adherence or infiltration into (peri)cardiac tissue. EUS is helpful in making the decision on whether to pursue a curative or a palliative therapeutic approach.

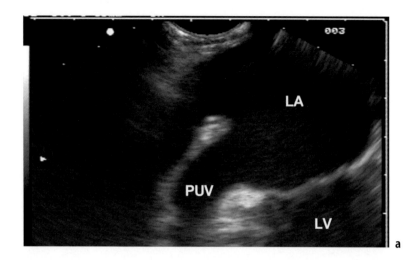

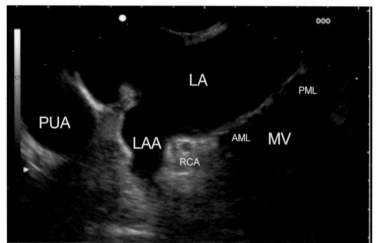

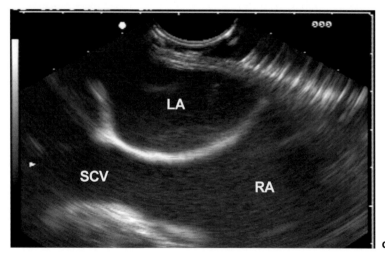

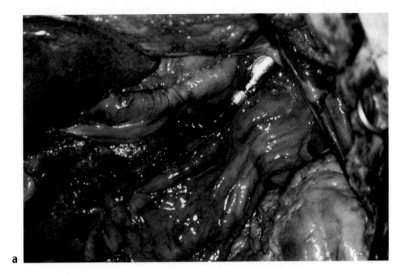

a

A view of the heart

Fig. 4.13 a–c. Right ventricle/Left ventricle: A view of the right (*RV*) and left ventricle (*LV*) can be depicted by advancing the endoscope into the gastric fundus and angulating the tip ventraly. The scanning plane is directed from below through the left lobe of the liver (*L*) into the mediastinum demonstrating the beating heart. The different muscle diameters of the ventricles are visible with a slight rotation. The reflex of the diaphragm (*DIA*) is visible as a hyperechoic border echo between the mediastinum and the abdomen. **a)** Simulation of the corresponding position of the EUS transducer in the stomach.

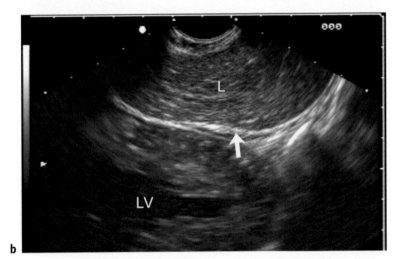

b

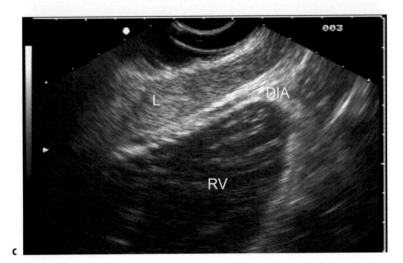

c

U. Will

CHAPTER 5
The Stomach and Paragastric Region: Imaging Techniques

(For abbreviations see page 175)

Note

If the transducer is directed *ventrally*, the scanning plane in the body moves with the direction of the rotation (right rotation moves the transducer to the right side of the body).

If the transducer is *dorsally* directed, the scanning plane moves in the opposite direction (right rotation moves the transducer to the left side of the body).

Your first landmark:
The aorta and the visceral vessels

1. Place the transducer in a longitudinal axis and rotate it until you see the typical formation of the aorta in front of the spine and follow the descending aorta.
2. The aorta should always be kept within the scanning field by maintaining the contact of the transducer with the dorsal gastric wall.
3. Below the cardia one can easily find the origins of the celiac trunk and the superior mesenteric artery. The hypoechoic insertion of the diaphragm is located ventrally to the aorta.
4. Keep the visceral arteries in your ultrasound-image and rotate the transducer to the right and you will guide the section plane of the abdomen to the left. This allows you to follow the pancreas from the body to the tail by withdrawing the instrument slowly.
5. Two vessels will follow your path:
   - the splenic artery.
   - the splenic vein, originating from the splenoportal confluence.
6. Try to get a section of the pancreas and demonstrate the pancreatic duct within the parenchyma.

Your second landmark:
The left kidney and the spleen

7. The upper pole of the left kidney is seen by following the pancreatic tail and withdrawing the transducer slowly.
8. Search for the renal hilum and demonstrate the renal artery and vein with a slow rotation to the left until you reach your first landmark: the aorta.

9. Turn back to the right and angulate the echoendoscope, following the splenic artery and vein into the splenic hilum.

Your third landmark: The splenoportal confluence and the head of the pancreas

10. Rotate back to the left and follow the splenic vein into the splenic confluence.
11. If you straighten the instrument in a longitudinal section through the confluence, you will find the superior mesenteric vein and with a slight rotation of the transducer to the left, you will see it course into the portal vein.
12. This section includes imaging of the pancreatic head surrounding the confluence and the superior mesenteric vein (uncinate process).
13. The common bile duct becomes visible behind the portal vein.

Your fourth landmark: The liver

14. Opposite to the aorta, rotate the instrument either to the right or to the left and you will find the left lobe of the liver with a guiding vessel: the left portal vein.
15. Try to follow the vessel with rotation until you see the portal vein, the biliary bifurcation and the portal hilum with the common bile duct and the common hepatic artery.
16. Further rotation will lead you to the hepatic veins and their confluence into the inferior vena cava.
17. Never forget to investigate the visible portions of the liver parenchyma.

Leaving the stomach on the way to the duodenum

18. You will be able to see the gallbladder with the tip of the transducer angled towards the head, while in a ventral orientation, on the way into the duodenum.
19. Inflate the stomach with air in order to pass from the pylorus into the duodenal bulb under endoscopic visualization.

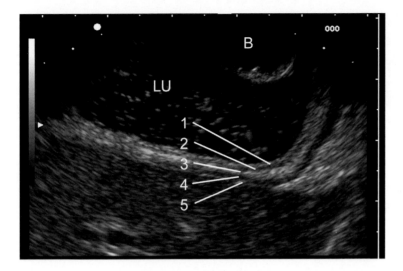

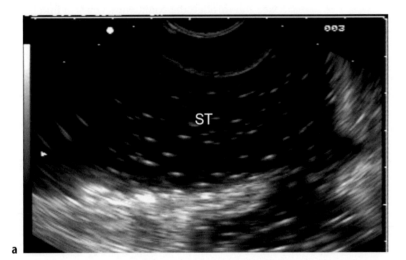

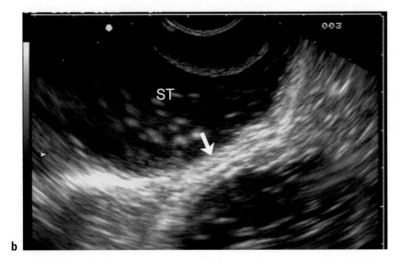

Fig. 5.1. Schematic image of the wall layers

Fig. 5.2 a, b. Normal gastric wall and angular fold: A systematic and total EUS examination of the stomach is not possible by using the longitudinal scanner. EUS examination is not required since EUS is only indicated for suspicious findings seen on standard upper endoscopy. In general, the tip of the endoscope is taken to the location of the lesion using an endoscopic view. There, the ballon is filled with water and the EUS transducer is coupled to the lesion and the surrounding tissue.

Exploring the stomach alone with the use of a ballon requires evacuation of insufflated endoluminal air, which results in to imaging artifacts. Subsequently, the stomach can be filled with water to optimize the coupling of the transducer with the gastric wall and to avoid artifacts caused by ballon-induced compression of the gastric wall. The subcardial region at the side of the fundus, the prepyloric region, and the angularis are often more difficult to identify. If there are problems in achieving sufficient ultrasound coupling due to lack of wave-mediating tissue, medium characteristics, or a lack of water, the patient's position should be changed so that the region of interest can be investigated by moving the water closer to the transducer. **(a, b)** A transverse section through the angularis reveals many layers, as a result of the angled stomach (ST) and the overlying gastric wall.

The first landmark: The aorta and the visceral arteries

Fig. 5.3. Aorta with the origin of the visceral arteries: Due to the longitudinal axis of the abdominal aorta, EUS can easily demonstrate the course of this vessel and its originating visceral arteries. The spine and the abdominal aorta become visible along with the origin of the celiac trunk and of the superior mesenteric artery after passing the cardia with a dorsally directed transducer. Close to the celiac trunk, a hypoechoic longitudinal structure reveals the median insertion of the diaphragm (diaphragmate hiatus of the aorta). These guiding structures are the main anatomical landmarks for the systematic EUS-investigation of the upper abdomen, and are important in the staging of esophageal and gastric carcinomas.

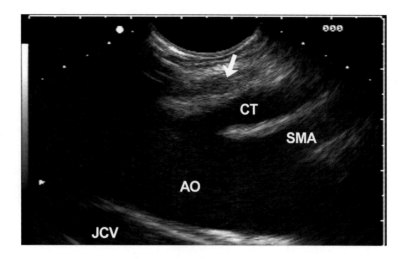

Fig. 5.4. Color Doppler endosonography of the celiac trunk and the superior mesenteric artery: The combination of color Doppler sonography and EUS provides numerous advantages in the abdomen. They facilitate orientation since the vessels may be more easily identified by their flow signals and pulsed Doppler spectrum. The orientation of the EUS transducer can be adjusted according to the course of the vessels. They are also used as landmarks for abdominal EUS.

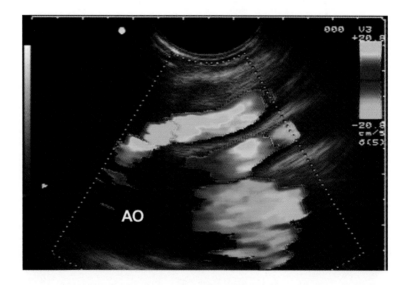

Fig. 5.5. Color power image of visceral arteries: Color power imaging Doppler sonography allows detection of low flow velocities which is not possible with conventional color Doppler sonography. In addition, the Doppler spectrum can reveal stenoses at the origins of the celiac trunk and the superior mesenteric artery. The figure shows the normal Doppler spectrum at the origin of the superior mesenteric artery.

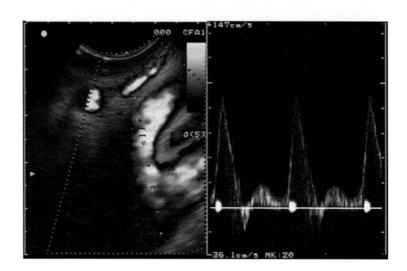

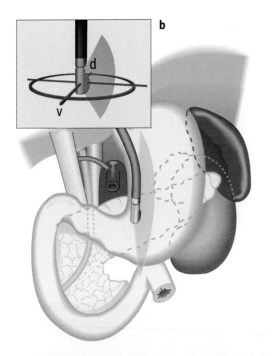

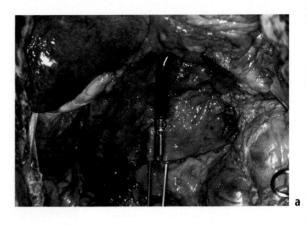

The second landmark: The pancreas, left kidney and spleen

Fig. 5.6 a–c. Body of the pancreas near the superior mesenteric artery: The investigator can observe numerous tubular structures in a longitudinal section of the proximal abdominal aorta (*AO*) with the ultrasound section directed dorsally and the transducer straight. These structures are classified as follows: The splenic artery (*SA*), peripheral from its origin out of the celiac trunk, is shown with a transverse section at the left side of the image. Below the splenic artery, the splenic vein (*SV*) shows an oval configuration. These two vessels partially lie against the body of the pancreas (*P*), which is partially seen. The left renal vein (*REV*) is found inferior to the superior mesenteric artery (*SMA*). **a, b** Simulation of the corresponding position of the EUS tranducer in the stomach.

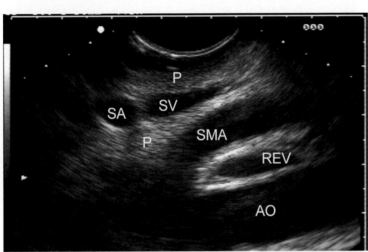

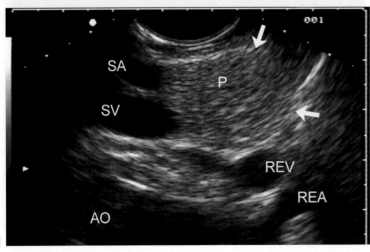

Fig. 5.6 d. Body of the pancreas: A slight rotation of the transducer to the right from the longitudinal view follows the course of the SA and SV and shows the main part of the pancreatic body. The flat contour of the pancreatic capsule is detectable and depicted as a dense border signal (*arrow*).

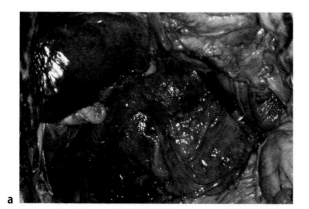

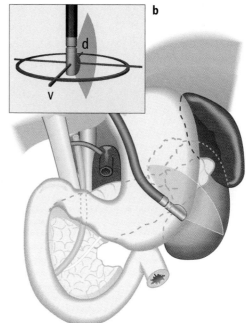

Fig. 5.7 a–d. Renal vessels and the tail of the pancreas: The endoscope is further rotated to the right and the transducer is slightly angulated to follow the vessels and to depict the tail of the pancreas. The extent of the angulation depends on the amount of depictable pancreatic parenchyma and the course of the vessels that serve as the guiding anatomic structures. The size and position of the tail of the pancreas varies. In a few cases, advancement of the instrument caudally is required (increasing the angulation) to keep the pancreas in the scanning plane. The picture demonstrates the close anatomic relationship between the pancreas and the left kidney (K). The renal hilum is almost visualized in a transverse section. The left artery of the kidney is dorsally located to the pancreas and can be followed from the aorta to the hilum. At the origin of the renal artery, pulsed Doppler can be applied. The course of the renal vein can be followed over the aorta from the hilum in the same way. **a, b** Simulation of the corresponding position of the EUS-transducer in the stomach.

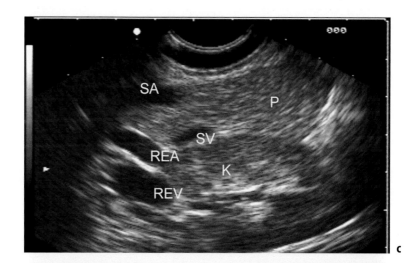

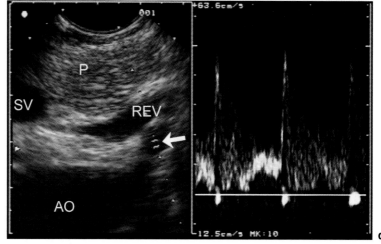

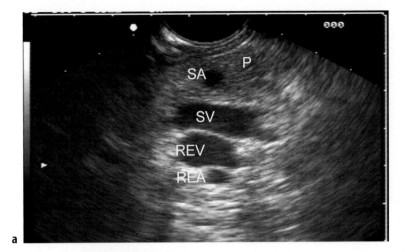

a

Fig. 5.8 a. Tail of the pancreas: It is necessary to rotate the transducer continuously to the right and to withdraw the instrument in order to view the full extent of the pancreatic body and tail. This maneuver is understandable if one realizes that the longitudinal axis of the pancreas lies transversely and is slightly cranially shifted in the upper retroperitoneal space. The splenic and renal vessels can be scanned in a cross-sectional plane in the same manner.

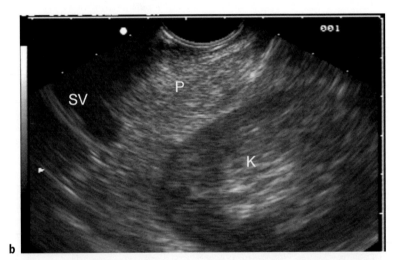

b

Fig. 5.8 b, c. Association between the left kidney and the tail of the pancreatic tail: The upper pole of the left kidney becomes visible dorsally to the pancreatic tail. If the angulation is slightly reduced, the ultrasound section of the pancreas changes. The pancreas now has a rhomboid form and the splenic vein is circular, indicating that both structures are represented in a longitudinal scan. The neighboring kidney is demonstrated with a different ultrasound section angle, resulting only in imaging of the hilum. The lower pole of the kidney is visualized infrequently.

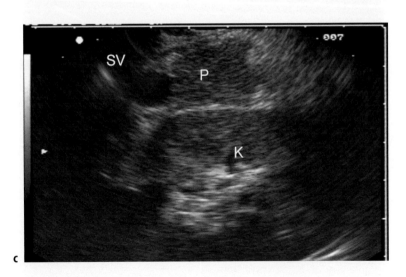

c

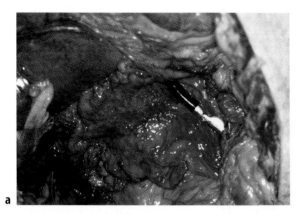

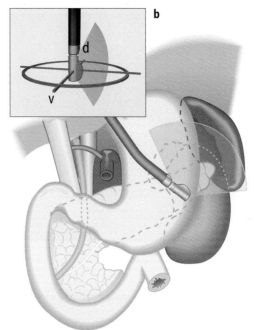

Fig. 5.9 a–d. Association between the tail of the pancreas and the spleen: The tail of the pancreas ends laterally near the splenic hilum. Therefore, further rotation of the transducer to the right along the pancreatic tail or the splenic vessels is necessary to reach the spleen. **a, b** Simulation of the corresponding position of the EUS transducer in the stomach.

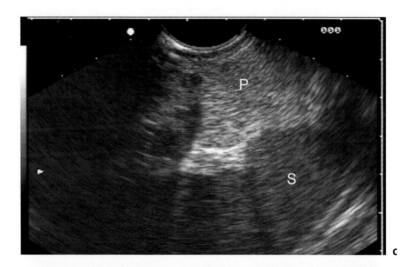

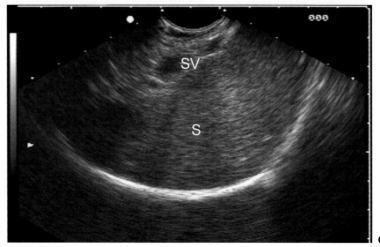

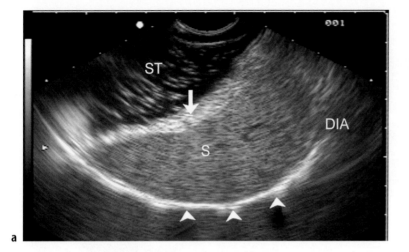

a

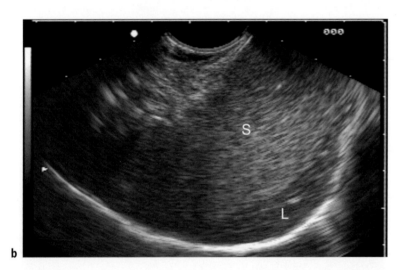

b

Fig. 5.10 a, b. Spleen: The pancreas disappears and the spleen becomes fully visible with continous rotation to the right and retraction of the scope. The spleen lies against the stomach along the posterior wall and along the greater curve **(a)**. The organ has a homogenous echopattern with only a few vessels and no bordering echoes. EUS investigation of the spleen and its parenchyma should be performed, if possible. The splenic hilum is also a region of interest in portal hypertension. **(b)** Turning the endoscope further to the right after depiction of a longitudinal section of the splenic hilum results in an oblique scanning plane directed ventrally. Using this ultrasound section, it is possible to image parts of the left lobe of the liver (*L*) below the left diaphragma by scanning through the spleen (*S*) if the liver extends to the far left side of the body.

Fig. 5.11 a–c. Left adrenal gland. The ultrasound section reaches the left adrenal gland (*AG*) after passing the upper pole of the kidney (*K*) by angling the EUS transducer to the left and withdrawing the endoscope. The kidney is considered, to along with the tail of the pancreas (*P*), as the guiding anatomic structure for finding the left adrenal gland, which lies behind the splenic vessels (*SV*) and the pancreas. The endosonographic morphology of the adrenal gland shows many variations. The most frequent one reveals an S-like configuration with a small central hyperechoic band (adrenal medulla) framed by a thin hypoechoic margin (adrenal cortex). **(a)** Simulation of the corresponding position of the EUS-transducer in the stomach.

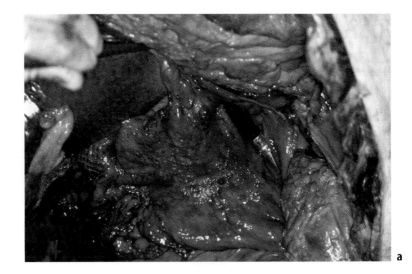

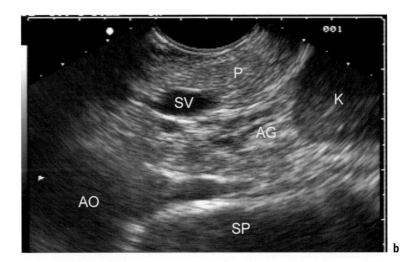

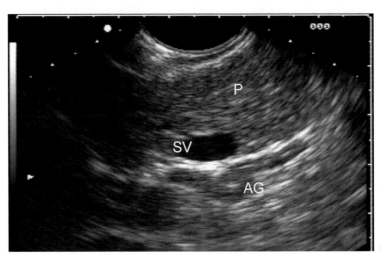

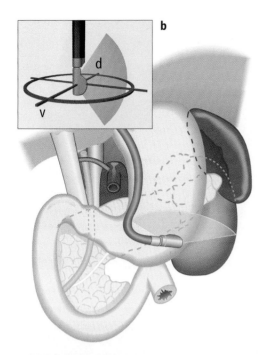

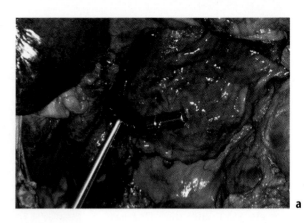

Fig. 5.12 a–d. Organ adapted section of the pancreas: Imaging the mesenteric vessels longitudinally, followed by dorsal angulation of the tip of the endoscope and rotation of the endoscope to the right leads to the visualization of a modified longitudinal ultrasound section of the pancreas. Centrally in the organ, the pancreatic duct becomes visible as a tubular formation with hyperechoic borders (*arrow*). Part of the tail of the pancreas can be seen at the bottom right of the figure. **a, b** Simulation of the corresponding position of the EUS transducer in the stomach. In Fig. 5.12 **c** the neighboring gastric wall shows a normal thickness with the typical five-layered structure (*arrowhead*). Due to the oblique scanning planes in Fig. 5.12 **d**, the gastric wall is shown with a varying thickness (*arrowheads*).

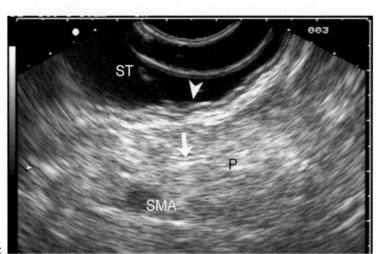

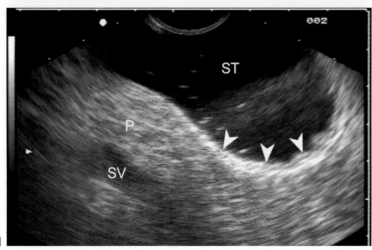

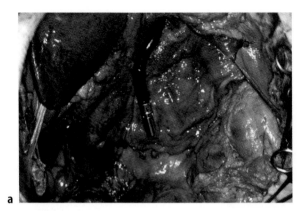

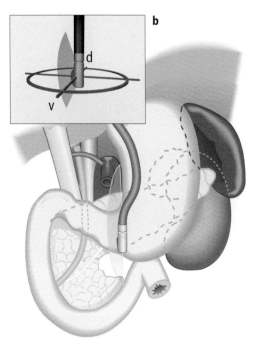

The third landmark:
The splenoportal confluence
and the head of the pancreas

Fig. 5.13 a–d. Head of the pancreas and confluence of the portal vein: The tip of the endoscope is positioned in the antrum or distal body of the stomach and is directed dorsally. The body of the pancreas (*P*) is depicted in a longitudinal section in front of the mesenteric vessels. Rotation of the endoscope to the left depicts the right part of the body and the proximal part of the head of the pancreas. Again, the vessels serve as guiding structures for anatomic orientation. The typical image of the confluence of the superior mesenteric vein and the splenic vein becomes visible and lead the investigator to the portal vein. The superior mesenteric artery (*SMA*) crosses along and to the left of the superior mesenteric vein (*SMV*). 5.13 **d** The normal pulsed Doppler spectra of the superior mesenteric vein. The venous flow spectrum can reveal portal hypertension, indicated by detection of backflow or a biphasic modulation. 5.13 **a, b** Simulation of the corresponding position of the EUS transducer in the stomach.

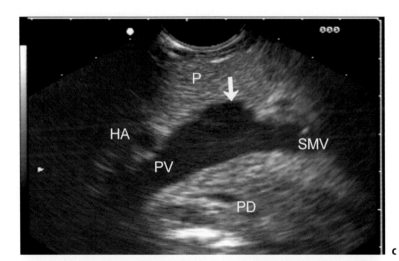

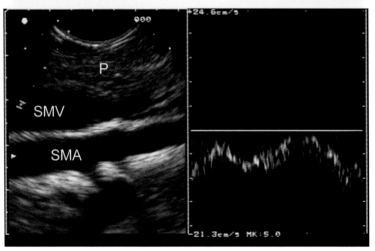

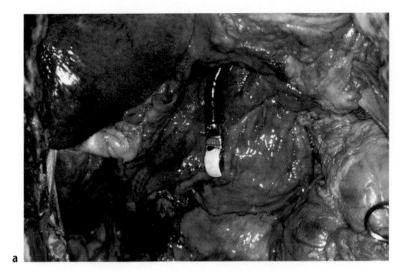

a

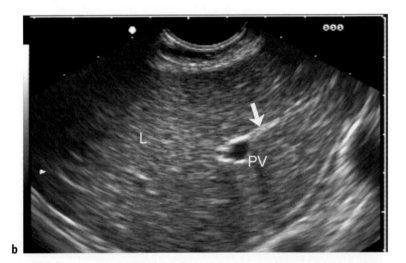

b

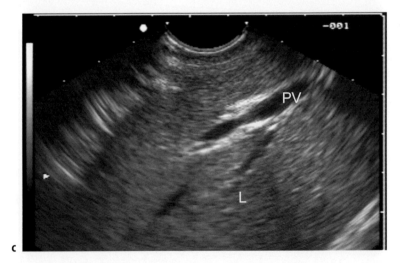

c

The fourth landmark: The liver

Fig. 5.14 a–c. Left lobe of the liver, ligamentum teres, and left branch of the portal vein: b) Continuing the rotation to the left allows depiction of the left lobe of the liver (*L*), which lies against the anterior wall of the stomach and is considered the anatomic guiding structure of this region. The correct ventral position is confirmed by the course of the ligamentum teres (*arrow*). Within this image, the left branch of the portal vein (*PV*) is shown in cross section, from which the ligamentum teres extends caudally and ventrally. **a)** Simulation of the corresponding position of the transducer in the stomach. **c)** The cross sectional plane of the left branch of the portal vein serves as a guiding anatomic structure to generate the image of the branches off the portal vein. The endoscope is rotated to the right and the tip is slightly angled. In addition, retraction or advancement of the endoscope can optimize the scanning plane to depict the left branch of the portal vein longitudinally. This branch can be a good guiding structure to search for the portal vein and the biliary bilar bifurcation.

Fig. 5.15 a–c. Hepatic veins: Withdrawing the endoscope along the left lobe of the liver (*L*) positions the EUS transducer back in the cardia. Directing the axially fixed EUS transducer to the right, the large-caliber hepatic veins become visible. **b)** The confluence of the three hepatic veins (right, middle, left) can be depicted by an image-adjusted angulation (anteflexion) of the tip of the EUS transducer. **c)** The hepatic veins can be followed, in part, into the periphery of the liver. Examination with color Doppler is helpful to locate and to follow the hepatic veins. **a)** Simulation of the corresponding position of the EUS transducer in the stomach.

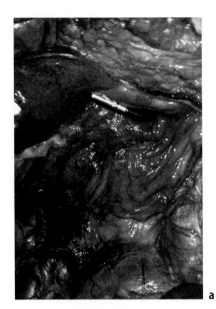

a

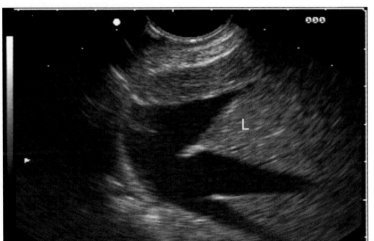

b

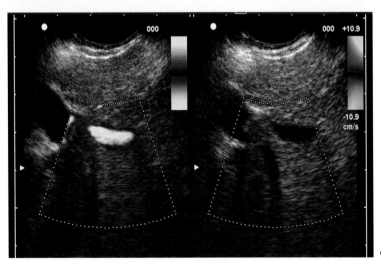

c

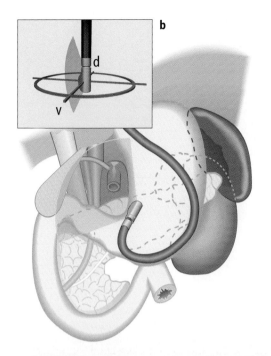

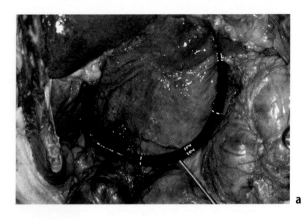

Leaving the stomach on the way to the duodenum

Fig. 5.16 a–d. Gallbladder: The gallbladder (*GB*) is closely situated to the gastric antrum and the duodenal bulb. Therefore, the EUS transducer must be positioned at least as far as the gastric antrum. Imaging of the gallbladder in this position is only possible if gastric air is completely evacuated and the tip of the transducer is pressed in a strongly angulated manner against the ventral wall of the antrum. If the gallbladder (*GB*) is depicted by this maneuver, the hepatoduodenal ligament, including the vascular structures, can be viewed by a slight additional rotation. The common bile duct (*arrow*), the hepatic artery (*HA*), and the portal vein (*PV*) are located right behind the gallbladder.

Incorporating color doppler and pulse Doppler sonography into this image allows the discrimination of the various tubular structures. **a, b)** Simulation of the corresponding position of the EUS transducer in the stomach.

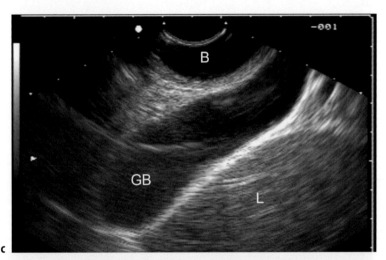

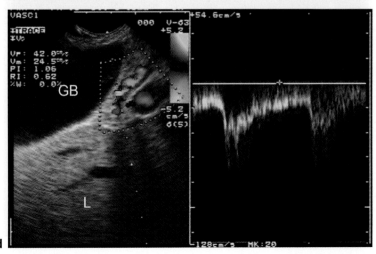

CHAPTER 6

The Duodenum and Pancreatobiliary System: Imaging Techniques

U. Will

(For abbreviations see page 175)

The Duodenum and pancreatobiliary system: Imaging techniques

1. After reaching the duodenal bulb, carefully pass by the tip of the bulb into the descending part of the duodenum with a rightward rotation.
2. Always straighten the echoendoscope after passing the duodenal bulb; otherwise, the instrument can induce pain and vomiting.
3. Fill the balloon in order to stabilize the instrument in the duodenum and to reduce the presence of surrounding air.
4. Search for the papilla with endoscopic or ultrasound visualization by carefully withdrawing the transducer.

Your first landmark: The pancreatic head and the mesenteric vessels

Withdrawing the instrument, you will get a lateral view of the pancreatic head and the mesenteric vessels (identified by color doppler).

Your second landmark: The pancreatic duct and the common bile duct

5. Withdraw the endoscope further until the papilla with the pancreatic and common bile ducts becomes visible.
6. Turn the instrument to the right in order to follow the pancreatic duct.
7. Then turn to the left, in order to follow the common bile duct (CBD) near the portal vein. Cranially to the CBD, the gastroduodenal artery becomes visible as a round vessel near the duodenal wall.
8. Remember that the (embryologically) ventral part often appears hypoechoic.
9. Be careful that the instrument does not dislodge or change position during rotation to the left.
10. Try to demonstrate the cystic duct and the gallbladder from this position.
11. Retract the endoscope into the duodenal bulb and find the gallbladder. By rotating, it may be possible to demonstrate the upper pole of the right kidney as well as the right adrenal gland.
12. Do not forget to deflate the balloon before passing the pylorus into the stomach, as this maneuver with a filled ballon is painful and involves the risk of ballon detachment.

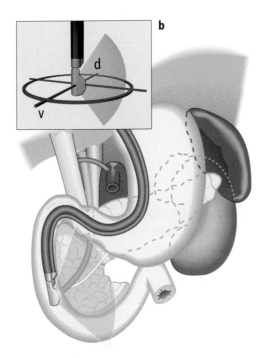

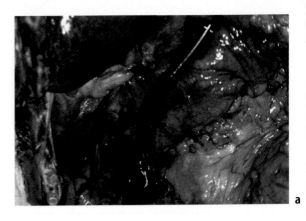

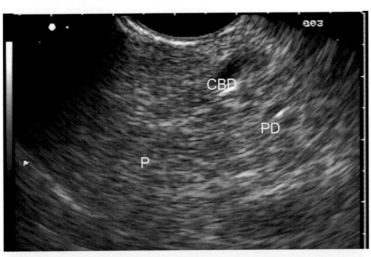

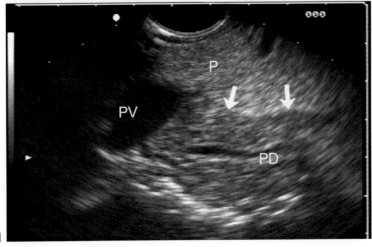

The first landmark:
The pancreatic head

Fig. 6.1 a–d. Descending duodenum/head of the pancreas: The transducer is inserted in the duodenum using the endoscopic view. After passing the tip of the duodenal bulb, the endoscope is straightened with a rightward rotation. Then, the papilla can be found either endoscopically or by ultrasound using the water filled balloon. The peripapillary region, along with the prepapillary parts of the pancreas (*PD*) and the common bile duct (*CBD*), serve as landmarks in the duodenum (**c**). The ventral part of the pancreas often appears as a hypoechoic and homogenous area. The fusion line where the ventral and dorsal parts of the pancreas are joined (*arrows*) is clearly visible (**d**). **a, b** Simulation of the corresponding position of the EUS transducer in the lumen.

**The second landmark:
The pancreatic duct
and the common bile duct**

Fig. 6.2 a–c. Prepapillary region: It should be easy to catch two small ellipsoid structures at the duodenal wall, which are the distal (intrapancreatic) of the biliary (*CBD*) and pancreatic ducts (*PD*). This is done by keeping the lateral orientation of the transducer while straightening the endoscope.

The distal parts of the ducts are better imaged by longitudinal sections, depending on the course of these ducts. Visualization is achieved by a slight elevation of the tip of the endoscope and by a rotation of the instrument to the left. By pushing or withdrawing the endoscope, it is possible to follow the ducts separately due to their different courses.

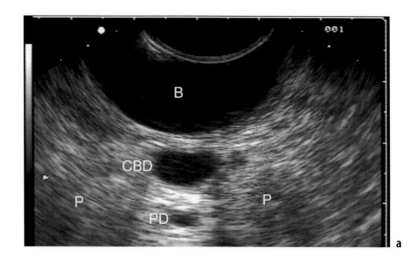

a

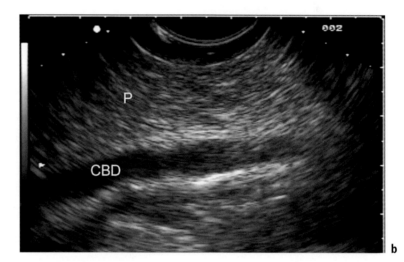

b

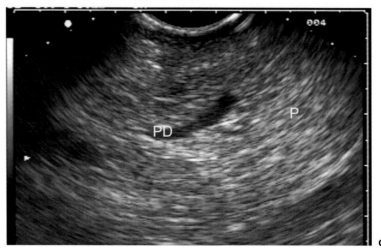

c

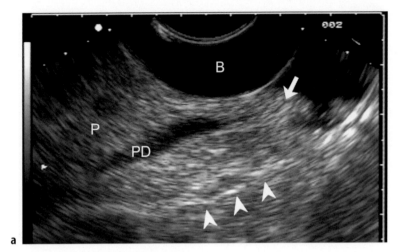

Fig. 6.3 a–c. Region of the papilla: The papilla is sometimes recognized as a polypoid prominence with thickening of the duodenal wall (*arrow*). The proximity of the pancreas to the right kidney (*K*) and inferior vena cava (*JCV*) is shown.

The pancreatic duct (*PD*), is seen within the head of the pancreas. The dorsal pancreatic capsule is depicted as a bordering reflex with a hyperechoic signal pattern (*arrowheads*). In Fig. 6.3**c**, the duodenal wall (*arrow*) with the regular five layered structure is seen near the prepapillary region.

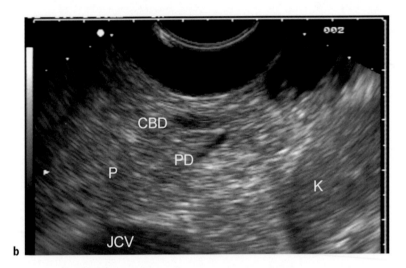

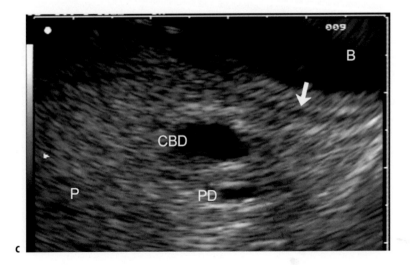

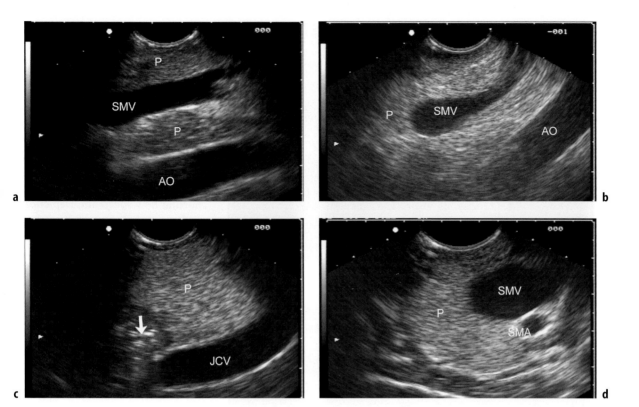

Fig. 6.4 a–d. Sequential images of the periduodenal structures from the duodenal bulb: a) The simplest visualization technique is the dorsally directed longitudinal ultrasound section through the head of the pancreas, from which all further steps are generated. The pancreas is scanned longitudinally and divided into two parts by the superior mesenteric vein. The dorsal part, situated between this vein and the aorta, is the uncinate process. The ventral part is the pancreatic isthmus. The aorta and the superior mesenteric vein are considered the anatomic guiding structures in this image. **b)** Rotating the endoscope slightly to the left results in depiction of the part of the pancreatic head that is situated to the right of the superior mesenteric vein. The seemingly divided parts of the head of the pancreas shown in the previous figure show a fusion, and the proximal segments of both the superior mesenteric vein and the aorta disappear from the scanning plane. Further rotation to the left moves the scanning plane through the head of the pancreas, which borders dorsally at the inferior vena cava (*JCV*). **c)** In front of this vein, the duodenum (*arrow*) is scanned transversely and indicated by central, air-induced reflexes. A slight advancement increases the transducer angulation, and the head of the pancreas is shown in a longitudinal section **(d)**. All the previous descriptions are based on a longitudinal fixation of the tip of the endoscope. These ultrasound sections show the pancreas in a cross sectional plane. The endoscope is further straightened to finally position it horizontally to the pancreas to generate a section along the longitudinal axis of the pancreas. This has the disadvantage that the head of the pancreas is depicted on the right side of the image (distant to the EUS transducer), whereas the body of the pancreas is shown on the left (close to the EUS transducer). This image is inverted compared with transcutaneous ultrasound, and may confuse orientation (see Fig. 3.4. in Chapter 3).

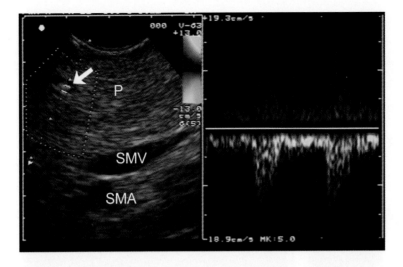

Fig. 6.5. Head of the pancreas/ gastroduodenal artery: Using the typical image of the head of the pancreas obtained from the duodenal bulb, a round anechoic structure, the gastroduodenal artery (*arrow*), is found at the upper margin of the pancreas. This vessel can be easily identified with color Doppler sonography. Pulsed Doppler sonography reveals a normal flow spectrum. Depiction and spectral analysis of this vessel can be used in the staging pancreatic carcinomas. Tumor infiltration into the artery can change flow characteristics.

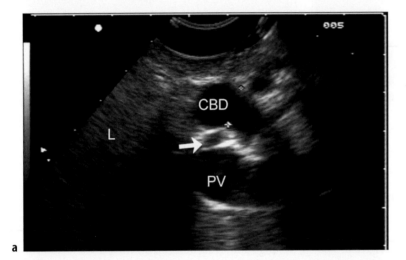

a

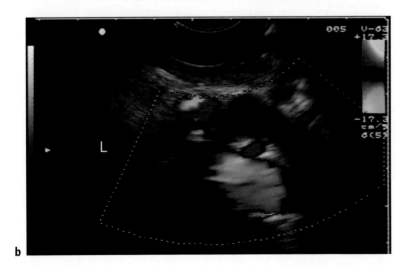

b

Fig. 6.6 a, b. Hepatoduodenal ligament: One of the most difficult maneuvers in EUS is obtaining an image of the hepatoduodenal ligament and its anatomic structures. Although it is relatively simple to depict the portal vein at its confluence, detection of the portal vein within the hepatoduodenal ligament up to the hepatic hilum is usually incomplete. A longitudinal image of the portal vein as the largest anatomic guiding structure of the hepatoduodenal ligament can be obtained by moving the tip of the endoscope to the left and keeping the initial direction dorsally. Subsequently, the EUS transducer is pressed (by a leftward rotation) onto the posterior wall of the duodenal bulb, allowing the transducer to be directed towards the liver (*L*). Using this position, the hepatic hilum can be imaged most of the time. Between the two tubular anechoic structures (closer to the EUS transducer: biliary duct (*CBD*); distant to the transducer: portal vein (*PV*)), the hepatic artery is seen in a transverse section (*arrow*). If there are difficulties in discriminating among these tubular structures, color doppler sonography can be used (**b**).

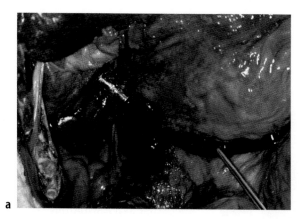

a

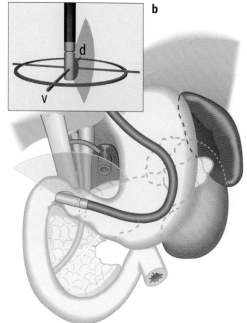

b

Fig. 6.7 a–d. Right adrenal gland:
The course of the pancreatic duct can be used to find the right adrenal gland (*AG*). An initially leftward-directed EUS transducer within the descending duodenum is elevated and subsequently the endoscope is turned to the left.
c) Hereby, the tip of the EUS scope is placed into a transverse position, with a dorsally directed EUS transducer. Thus, structures on the right side are depicted on the right side of the image (cranial part of the EUS transducer) (likewise for the left). Retaining this degree of angulation, the endoscope is retracted to the duodenal bulb and is slightly turned to the left. First the pancreas (*P*), and subsequently the right kidney (*K*), disappear from the scanning plane. The anatomic guiding structures are the aorta (*AO*) and the inferior vena cava (*JCV*).
d) Dorsally to the inferior vena cava, in front of the vertebral column (*SP*), a longitudinal structure is detected, which has a central hyperechoic focus (indicating the adrenal medulla) surrounded by a hypoechoic margin (adrenal cortex). **a, b)** Simulation of the corresponding position of the EUS transducer in the duodenal bulb.

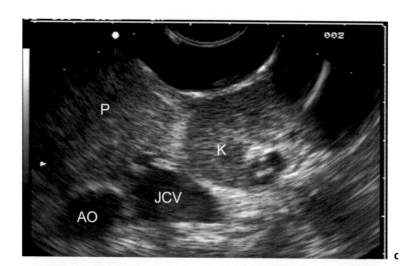

c

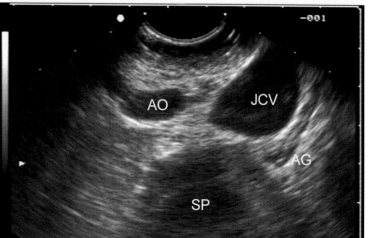

d

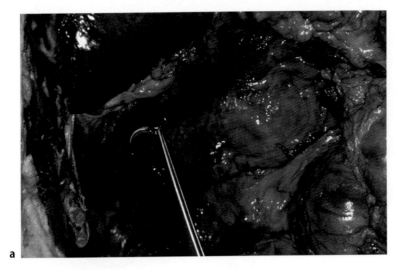

a

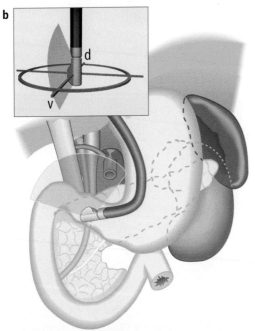

b

Fig. 6.8 a–c. Gallbladder visualization from the duodenal bulb: The gallbladder is situated against the front wall of the duodenal bulb and serves as the ventral landmark for EUS scanning planes obtained from the duodenal bulb. EUS investigation of the gallbladder from the duodenal bulb is possible by advancing the tip of endoscope when it is positioned in the antrum, or by straightening the endoscope as it is withdrawn from the descending duodenum. The latter option may disadvantageous in that the tip of the endoscope can easily dislocate out of the duodenal bulb backwards through the pylorus. This risk can be minimized by maximally filling the ballon with water. The EUS transducer is usually directed to the right lateral side of the duodenum. Therefore, the anterior wall of the gallbladder is depicted by rotating the endoscope to the left. A full image of the gallbladder is generated by further endoscope manipulations. **a, b)** Simulation of the corresponding position of the EUS transducer in the duodenal bulb.

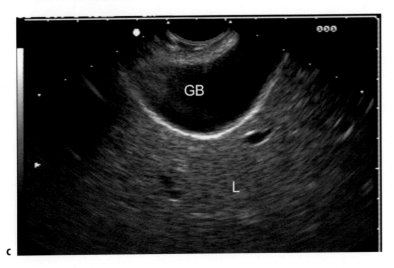

c

Fig. 6.9 a, b. Inferior vena cava: A longitudinal section along the inferior vena cava (*JCV*) from the descending duodenum, infrequently used in gastroenterology, can be obtained. The transducer is directed dorsally in accordance with the course of the duodenum. The close association between the inferior vena cava and the portal vein (*PV*) is shown. The portal vein appears at the upper margin of figure **b** with an oval configuration, which slightly narrows the inferior vena cava. Dorsally to the inferior vena cava, the right renal artery (*REA*) is demonstrated. Pulsed Doppler sonography reveals a regular low-resistance spectrum. The clinical value of EUS-based Doppler sonography for evaluation of renal artery blood flow has not yet been established.

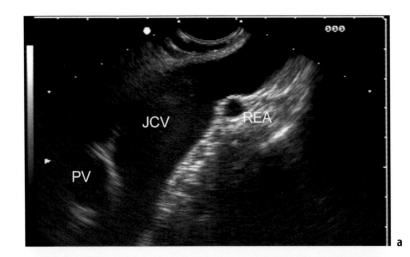

a

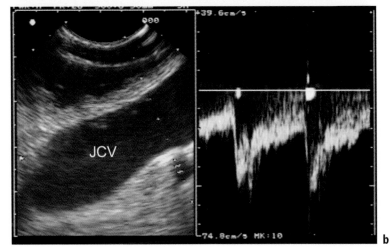

b

Final remarks

The periluminal structures from the esophagus, the stomach, and the duodenum as shown by EUS, were described. These instructions are intended as supportive guidelines for endosonographic beginners in obtaining and maintaining orientation during the EUS investigation.

With this description we do not claim completeness, and the suggested approaches and images should not be considered as the only options for depicting certain anatomic structures. Other investigators may have modified these steps to generate similar endosonographic images. Standardized images have been developed to facilitate systematic evaluation and allow for reproducibility. The successful longitudinal endosonographer can visualize and recognize the anatomic guiding structures or landmarks. This is a prerequisite for maneuvering between the complicated scanning planes in order to provide a complete EUS examination.

Acknowledgments

I would like to thank Mr. T. Fuchs, Mr. H. Bock, Mrs. M. Rau and Prof. Raabe for their support in the preparation and production of the photographs used in this chapter. I am grateful to R. Neumann, M.D., for providing the CT scans and P. Kann, M.D., for any helpful comments. I gratefully acknowledge the editorial assistance of F. Meyer, M.D., and Linda Kesselring, MS, ELS.

PART 3

Pathology

(For abbreviations see page 175)

E. Burmester · C. Jakobeit · L.Welp

J. Janssen · L. Greiner · P. Vilmann · U. Will

CHAPTER 7
Esophagus

(For abbreviations see page 175)

Fig. 7.1. Stage T1, adenocarcinoma. A small hypoechoic, well demarcated lesion of the distal esophagus is seen in the mucosa (*MM*). The submucosa is only partially infiltrated. The muscularis propria is intact. The short distance between the ultrasound transducer and the wall is due to compression by the balloon. A better image quality can be expected when the esophageal lumen is filled with water, but this can be risky (aspiration).

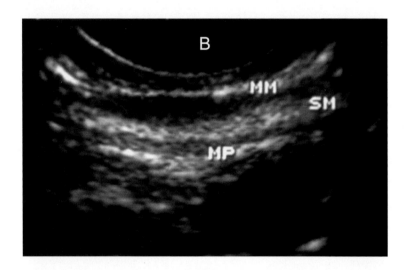

Fig. 7.2. Stage T1, esophageal carcinoma. This small squamous cell carcinoma of the esophagus infiltrates the mucosa and submucosa. The border between tumor and the sandwich-like muscularis propria is very narrow (*arrowheads*). Transducer pressure on the wall must be minimized in order to avoid overstaging. Slight movements with the transducer confirm the sliding of the submucosa over the muscularis propria. At this stage the standard treatment is surgery because of the enhanced risk of lymph node metastases.

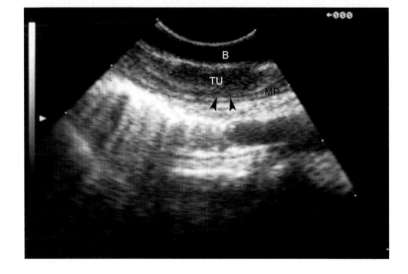

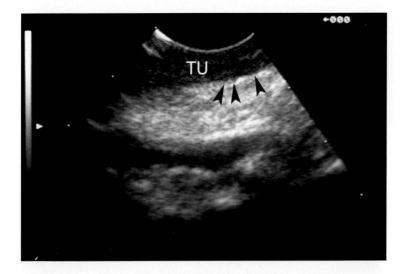

Fig. 7.3. Stage T2 esophageal carcinoma. Hypoechoic, transmural infiltration of all wall layers characterizes the T2 stage of esophageal cancer (*TU*). There are very small, hypoechoic indentations into the adventitia (*arrowhead*) that may represent an inflammatory reaction, possibly to be differentiated by real-time mode imaging. In some cases, more severe inflammation might lead to overstaging of the tumor.

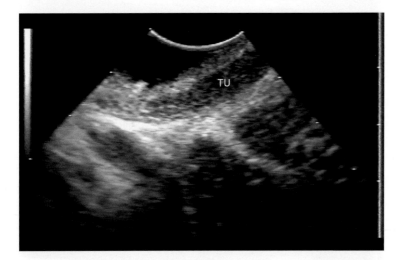

Fig. 7.4. Stage T2 esophageal carcinoma. The hypoechoic tumor (*TU*) is seen invading into the muscularis propria layer.

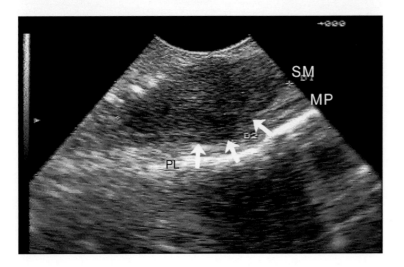

Fig. 7.5. Stage T3 squamous cell carcinoma. A stenotic, inhomogeneous, hypoechoic tumor which infiltrates and spreads locally beyond the muscularis propria (*arrows*) with an irregular outer margin is seen. The main tumor mass is located in the mucosa. The esophageal lumen is not visible due to compression by the balloon and no water in the lumen. With stenotic tumors, it can be especially risky to fill the lumen with water (aspiration).

Fig. 7.6. Stage T3 esophageal carcinoma. This esophageal carcinoma (*TU*) could not be traversed with the echoendoscope. Therefore the thickness of the tumor could not reliably be measured. Nevertheless, infiltration of the adventitia is clearly seen (*arrowhead*), indicating at least stage T3 carcinoma. The patient, who also had large paraesophageal lymph nodes, underwent combined radio-chemotherapy.

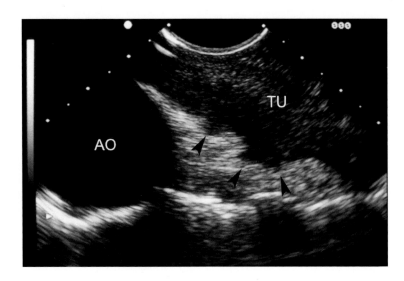

Fig. 7.7. Stage T4 esophageal carcinoma. This carcinoma of the esophagus is in close contact with the aortic wall at the aortic arch (*arrowheads*). Usually this finding necessitates palliative treatment only.

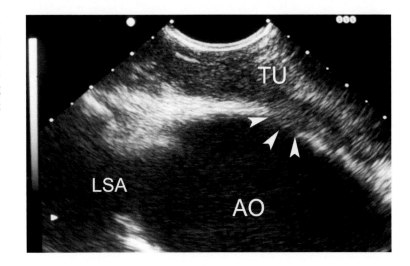

Fig. 7.8. Stage T4 carcinoma. A large stenotic, non-traversable tumor with widespread infiltration of the esophageal wall into the paresophageal fat tissue and the aorta is seen. Nodular tumor masses in the aortic lumen are seen (*arrows*). A complete loss of the esophageal layer structure due to hypoechoic tumor masses and ulceration with air artifacts is seen (*arrowheads*). Failure to traverse the stenosis allows only an investigation of the proximal tumor margin and may be not sufficient for T and N staging.

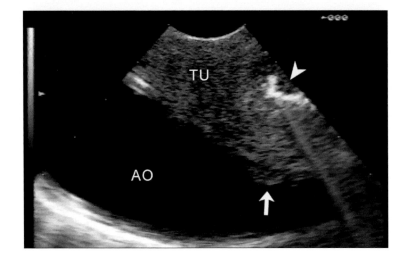

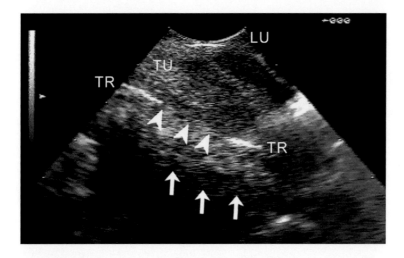

Fig. 7.9. Stage T4 squamous cell carcinoma. A stenotic tumor (*TU*) with penetration into the trachea (*TR*) is seen. The pearl-string like, hyperechoic line of the tracheal wall is interrupted by the tumor (*arrowheads*). Typical artifacts in the trachea induced by air are visualized (*arrows*). Only a small part of the esophageal lumen (*LU*) is visible due to complete compression of the balloon by the stenosis.

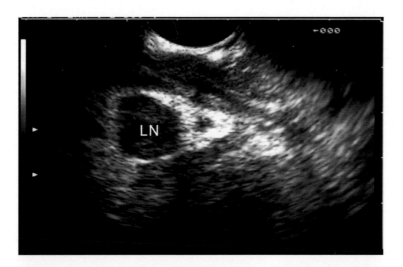

Fig. 7.10. Stage T3N1 esophageal cancer. A hyperechoic tumor with a 1.5-cm lymph node (*LN*) is seen immediately below the transducer. The lymph node is hyperechoic and round with distinct borders.

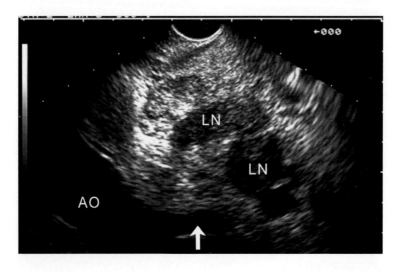

Fig. 7.11. (Stage M1a). Esophageal cancer with distant lymph node metastases. Multiple hypoechoic lymph nodes are located around the celiac axis. *AO*, Aorta; *arrow*, celiac axis; *LN*, lymph nodes.

Fig. 7.12. Stage M1a esophageal cancer. A large lymph node metastasis at the celiac axis is seen. Infiltration of the splenic artery and vein is present. There are irregular boundaries of the tumor and a missing interface between the vessel and the tumor (*arrows*). The diagnosis of tumor infiltration was confirmed by fine-needle aspiration. The color Doppler is helpful in visualizing the vessels before FNA.

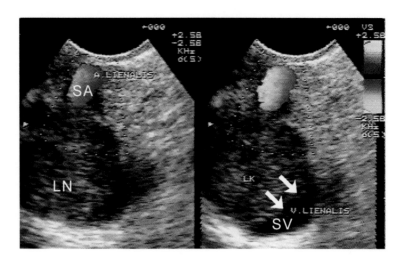

Fig. 7.13. Gastroesophageal reflux disease (GERD). This image shows hypoechoic thickening of the mucosa and a very narrow submucosal layer in a patient with severe reflux esophagitis. The EUS aspect is the same as in mucosal-type T1 carcinoma. The final diagnosis can only be made by endoscopic biopsies and subsequent follow-up, with repeated biopsy if necessary.

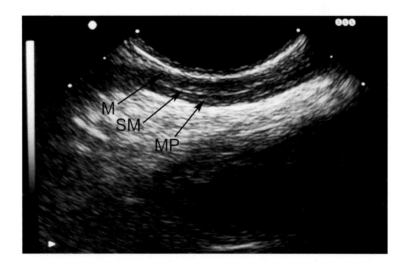

Fig. 7.14. Peptic stenosis in GERD: stenosis at the level of the lower esophagus. The balloon is compressed and the mucosa shows a hypoechoic, inflammatory infiltration with a nearly normal submucosa and an intact muscularis propria. Differentiation from a T1 carcinoma is difficult or even impossible. EUS has a low accuracy in differentiating between malignant and inflammatory changes. Histological confirmation is always necessary, especially in patients with Barrett's esophagus.

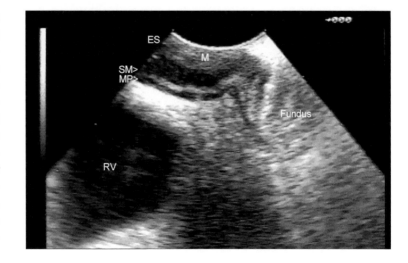

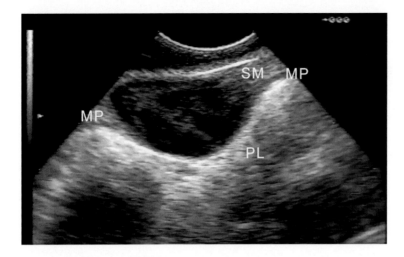

Fig. 7.15. Leiomyoma of the esophagus originating in the fourth layer, corresponding to the muscularis propria. Submucosal tumors of the upper gastrointestinal tract are one of the main indications for EUS. Leiomyomas are usually homogeneous and hypoechoic and develop from the second or fourth layer. This case is an example of a cyst-like tumor with a nearly anechoic pattern due to necrosis. Only a few echoes are visible in the center.

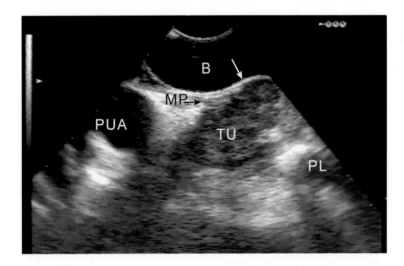

Fig. 7.16. Leiomyosarcoma. A predominantly submucosally spreading, large, hypoechoic tumor in the middle part of the esophagus with irregular margins and nodular boundaries is seen originating in the fourth layer. Note the intact first layer (*arrow*) in correlation with the endoscopic aspect of a submucosal tumor. The echo pattern of there tumors is usually inhomogeneously hypochoic. In the case of necrosis, anechoic areas may be possible. Even hyperechoic foci due to hyaline degeneration may be seen.

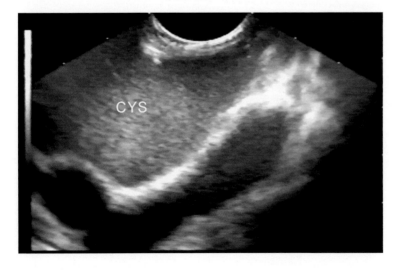

Fig. 7.17. A large **intramural esophageal cyst** with echogenic material inside the cyst; compression of the heart is seen.

Fig. 7.18. Esophageal varices. Intramural varices of the distal esophagus are visualized by color Doppler. *Arrows,* Outer margin of the esophageal wall.

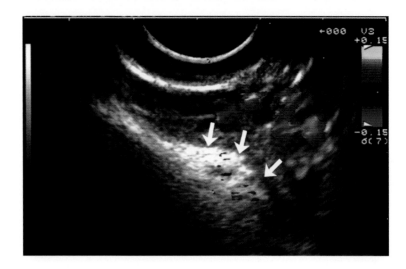

Fig. 7.19. Fundic varices. Typical intramural varices in a patient with liver cirrhosis and portal hypertension. Tortuous vessels appearing as multiple round and oval, anechoic areas in the submucosa are seen. EUS is superior to endoscopy in demonstrating gastric submucosal vessels. EUS is helpful in the differential diagnosis between varices and large gastric folds. Color Doppler can easily demonstrate blood-flow.

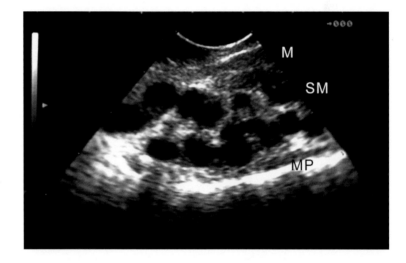

Fig. 7.20. Esophageal varix after sclerotherapy. The broad hypoechoic transformation of the mucosa of the esophageal wall is caused by thrombosis of a subepithelial varix after sclerotherapy (*arrowheads*). The neighboring layers show an inflammatory reaction with infiltration of the adventitia (*arrows*). In cases of a nearly anechoic thrombosis, color Doppler EUS may help to decide whether there still is some residual perfusion within the varix.

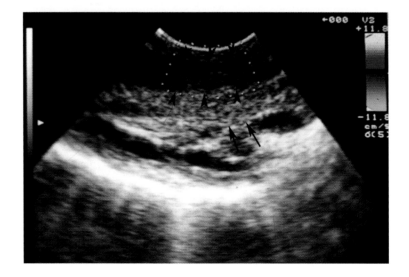

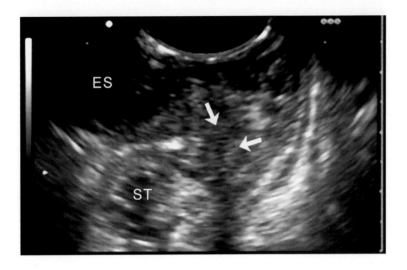

Fig. 7.21. Achalasia. The water-filled esophagus appears to be dilated, while a concentric thickening of the wall (*arrows*) is found at the cardia. All layers, especially on the right side, are detectable, and the outer margin is smooth. The gastric fundus has a normal wall without signs of tumor infiltration, as seen in "pseudo"-achalasia, which results from carcinoma of the cardia. However, these two entities cannot be distinguished reliably by EUS.

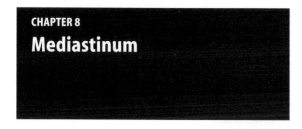

CHAPTER 8
Mediastinum

E. Burmester · J.-U. Erk · J. Janssen · L. Greiner

P. Vilmann · U. Will · M. Wittenberg

(For abbreviations see page 175)

Fig. 8.1. Extraluminal compression of the esophagus by the aorta. A pulsating tumor and suspected submucosal tumor were seen on esophagoscopy. Color Doppler EUS clearly identifies the "tumor" as an impression by the aortic arch (*AO*). Note that the normal esophageal wall (*arrows*) can be followed overlying the vessel and that it is demarcated by a small, light border between the wall and the vessel. EUS is highly accurate (94%) in differentiating submucosal tumors from extraluminal compression.

Fig. 8.2. Aneurysm of the thoracic aorta. Aneurysms and dissections of the thoracic aorta (*AO*) are seen only occasionally in gastroenterological endosonography. Nevertheless, the gastroenterologist should be familiar with these findings, which can be visualized by longitudinal EUS. This aneurysm of the thoracic aorta with a diameter of 5.5 cm was diagnosed by chance during EUS. Close to the aortic arch a saccular expansion with an excavated thrombus (*arrowheads*) is seen.

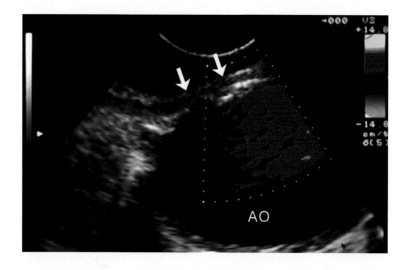

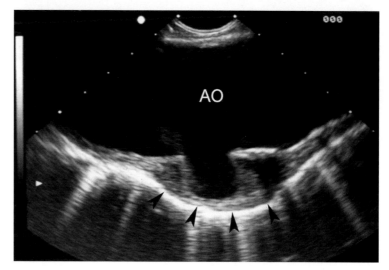

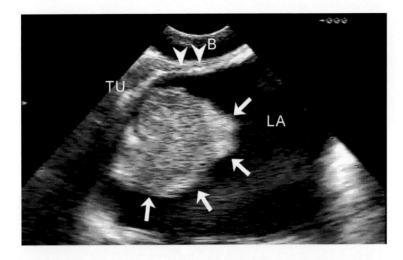

Fig. 8.3. Thrombus in the left atrium: an accidental finding of a thrombus in the left atrium (*arrows*) during EUS staging of a cardia carcinoma. The thrombus is floating in the lumen and adherent to the wall. Investigation with 5 MHz allows very deep penetration and demonstration of the adjacent organs in the mediastinum. The normal esophageal wall (*arrowheads*) and parts of the infiltrated cardia are seen between the balloon and the pericardium.

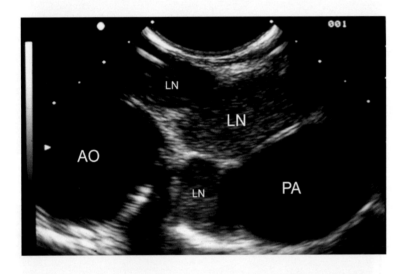

Fig. 8.4. Lymph node metastases in the aortopulmonary window. The aortopulmonary window with the pulmonary artery can be inspected well by longitudinal EUS. Small lymph nodes of about 3–5 mm are nearly always found, whereas enlarged hypoechoic nodes as in this figure are pathological. EUS guided fine-needle aspiration biopsy can be easily carried out if necessary. In this case, the node enlargement resulted from metastatic non-small cell lung cancer.

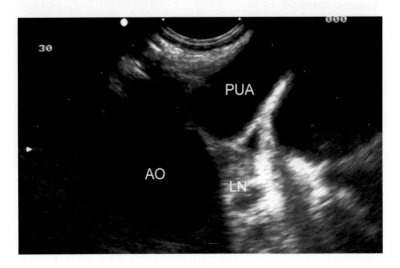

Fig. 8.5. Metastatic lymph node (diameter 18×15 mm) between the ascending aorta and the main stem of the pulmonary artery in a patient with an adenocarcinoma of the left upper lobe. Possible signs of malignancy are a sharp border, round shape, and a diameter of more than 10 mm (15 mm in the subcarinal region). The internal echoes are unusual in that they are rather echogenic. An invasion of the surrounding vessels is not present.

Fig. 8.6. Lymph node at the tracheal bifurcation. Sagittal section of the lower part of the trachea with a homogeneous hypoechoic lymph node 7 mm in diameter. Further diagnostic procedures including EUS guided aspiration needle biopsy showed no sign of malignancy.

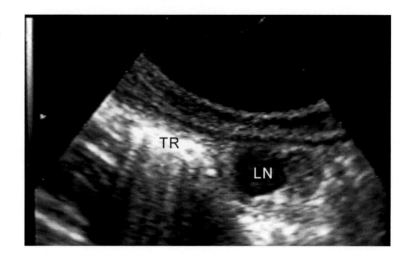

Fig. 8.7. Mesothelioma of the pleura. The transducer is placed against the esophageal wall. A longitudinal hypoechoic lesion is located close to the esophagus. Color Doppler flow in a vessel is visualized adjacent to the lesion. *Arrows*, reflexions from an air filled lung.

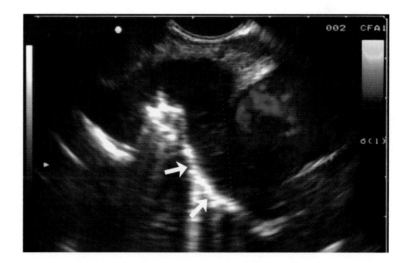

Fig. 8.8. Pulmonary cancer of the right lung. An hypoechoic lesion (*TU*) is located adjacent to the esophagus at the right lung hilum. *Arrow*, reflexions from air-filled lung tissue.

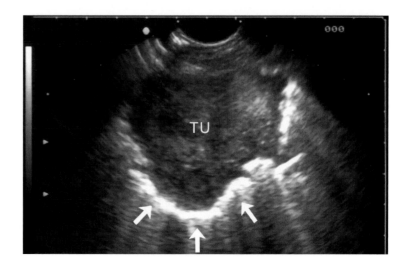

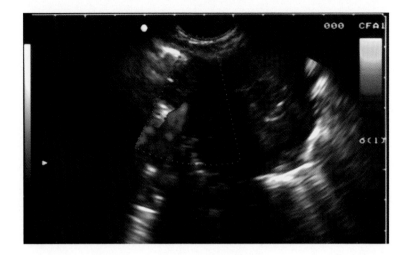

Fig. 8.9. Cancer of the right lung. This image is taken from the same patient as in Fig. 8.8. A power Doppler image is seen adjacent to the (hypoechoic) lung tumor.

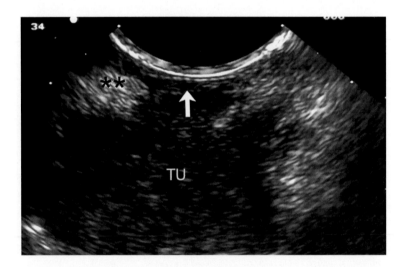

Fig. 8.10. Invasion of a locally advanced lung cancer into the esophagus (confirmed by thoracotomy). The hyperechoic layer (*asterisks*) notes the tissue between the esophageal wall and the tumor. In the middle of the image the hypoechoic tumor (*TU*) invades the muscularis propria (arrow).

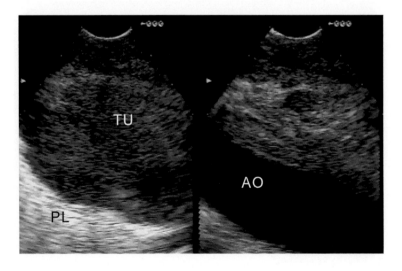

Fig. 8.11. Lymph node infiltration in non-Hodgkins lymphoma. A large, hypoechoic, inhomogeneous mediastinal mass is seen surrounding the aorta and compressing the lung. Note that the border of the tumor (*TU*) is poorly visualized. Differentiation between lymphoma and metastatic lymph nodes in carcinoma is not possible by EUS. *AO* = aorta

Fig. 8.12. Bronchial cyst. In the middle esophagus, a cystic formation is seen between the esophageal wall and the lung. The cyst shows some hyperechoic reflections and sediment (*arrow*). The esophageal lumen is compressed by the cyst. The air-induced reverberation echoes mark the margin of the cyst and reveal adherence to the lung (*arrowheads*). The sediment indicates that the cyst may be infected. This was confirmed by EUS guided fine-needle aspiration and subsequent microbiological culture of the fluid.

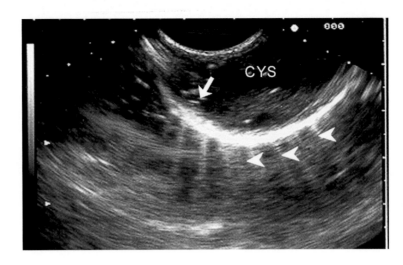

Fig. 8.13. Lung cancer of the right upper lobe with corresponding poststenotic atelectasis. The entire upper region is filled by an hypoechoic lesion with a slightly inhomogeneous internal echo. Doppler EUS helps to characterize the central vessels which mark the border between the tumor and the collapsed lung (*asterisks*).

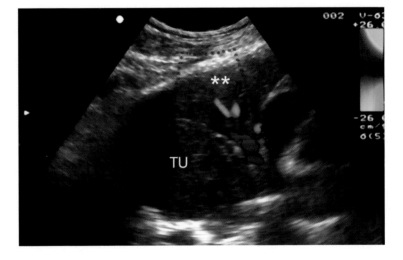

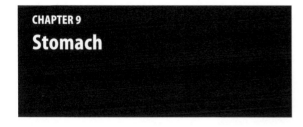

CHAPTER 9
Stomach

E. Burmester · J.-U. Erk · C. Jakobeit

J. Janssen and L. Greiner · P. Vilmann · U. Will

(For abbreviations see page 175)

Fig. 9.1. Adenocarcinoma in stage T1. A very small polypoid tumor (*between the markers ++*) is seen in the corpus of the stomach with hypoechoic pattern invading the lamina propria and the submucosa. The muscularis propria is intact. To visualize this small lesion a water filling to generate an interface between the balloon and the wall and an adequate distance between wall and transducer are absolutely necessary. *LU* Water-filled lumen.

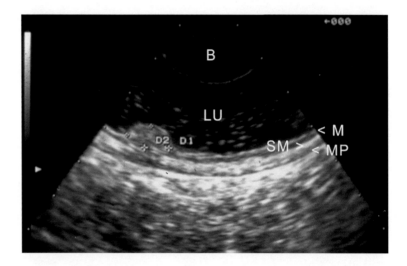

Fig. 9.2. Early gastric cancer in stage T1. An hypoechoic lesion invading the superficial part of the submucosal layer can be seen. The five wall layers of the stomach are clearly seen.

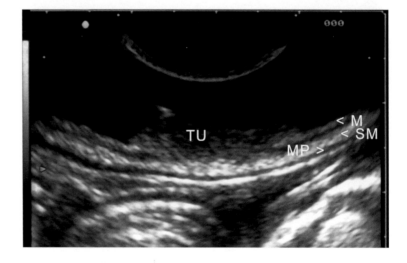

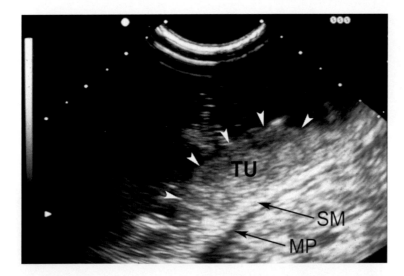

Fig. 9.3. Gastric carcinoma in stage T1. This exophytic gastric carcinoma is characterized by mucosal thickening (*arrowhead*). Due to comorbidity and the T1 stage, the patient was selected for endoscopic therapy. Histologically small tumor islands were seen within the submucosa, which could not be detected by EUS. Patients in better clinical condition would have to undergo subsequent surgery because of the enhanced risk of lymph node metastases.

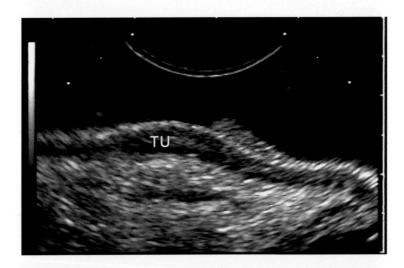

Fig. 9.4. Gastric carcinoma in stage T1. Hypoechoic tumor infiltrating the mucosa.

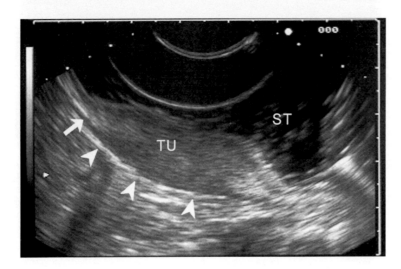

Fig. 9.5. Gastric carcinoma in stage T2N0. The gastric tumor, located at the greater curvature, shows a hypoechoic, homogeneous signal pattern. Discrimination of the muscularis propria (*arrow*) is not possible in the tumor area. Only the fifth layer, the serosa, is seen as a smooth hyperechoic outline (*arrowheads*). *Left*, near the tumor, all five layers can be differentiated. The stomach has been filled with water, providing better acoustic coupling of the ultrasound waves to the tumor.

Fig. 9.6. Adenocarcinoma in stage T2. EUS section through the angular fold. The investigation of the angular fold requires a sufficient fluid interface between the transducer and the wall, but it is sometimes difficult to achieve in this region. The tumor is directly located in the fold with the main tumor masses in the submucosa infiltrating the muscularis propria but not interrupting the outer margin. *LU*, Water-filled lumen

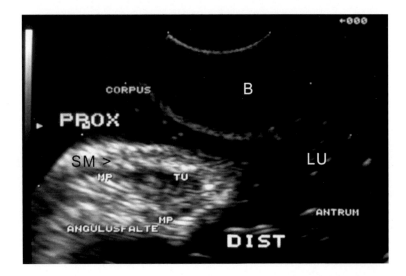

Fig. 9.7. Gastric carcinoma in stage T2N1. This malignant ulcer shows transmural hypoechoic infiltration. The outer border must be carefully inspected to determine invasion beyond the serosa (*arrowheads*). The differentiation between tumor invasion into the subserosa, as in this case (stage T2), or beyond the serosa (stage T3) by EUS remains problematic. The hypoechoic round lymph node of 1 cm is suspected to have metastatic infiltration, which was confirmed histologically. However, the morphological criteria to define malignant versus benign remain ambiguous.

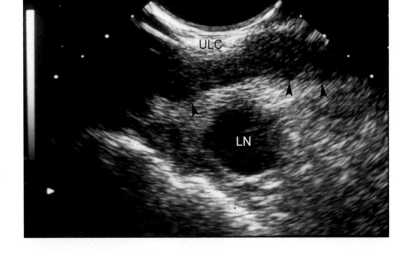

Fig. 9.8. Gastric carcinoma in stage T2. The endosonographic image shows tumor infiltration into the submucosa and muscularis propria.

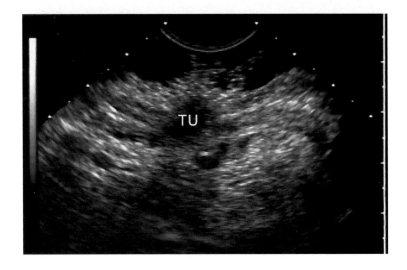

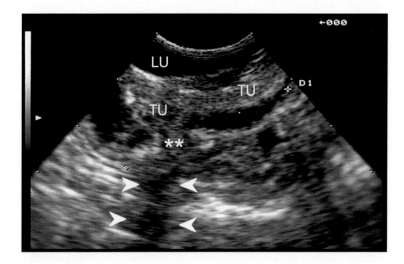

Fig. 9.9. Adenocarcinoma in stage T3. Transmural infiltration of the gastric wall with, complete destruction of the layers and hypoechoic thickening of the muscularis propria and penetration into the serosa (*asterisks*). *Left*, a normal gastric wall with the typical layer structure. The shadow (*arrowheads*) between normal and pathological layer structure is due to air bubbles in the gastric mucus. *LU*, Water-filled stomach lumen

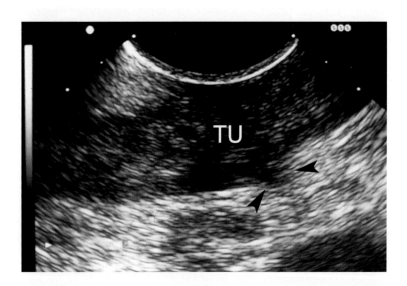

Fig. 9.10. Gastric carcinoma in stage T3. This gastric carcinoma infiltrates the entire gastric wall and locally penetrates the serosa (*arrowhead*), indicating a stage T3 carcinoma.

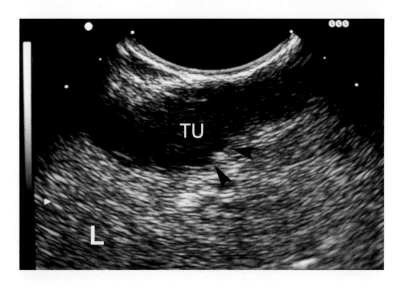

Fig. 9.11. Gastric carcinoma in stage pT4. EUS of the lesser curvature shows a large hypoechoic tumor that invades the left liver lobe (*arrowhead*). Movement of the transducer confirmed the fixation of the tumor to the liver. This finding was confirmed at the time of surgery.

Fig. 9.12. Gastric cancer in stage T4. The transducer is placed against an hypoechoic lesion (*TU*) that has completely destroyed the normal wall layer structure in the gastric body. Deep penetration of tumor tissue with invasion into the pancreatic body (*P*) is seen in the center of the image. The tumor is in close contact with the pancreatic duct (*PD*).

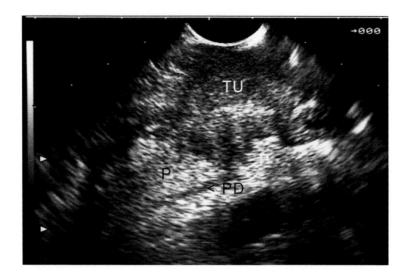

Fig. 9.13. Adenocarcinoma of the anastomosis (histopathologic stage T1) after Bilroth II resection in 1960. The tumor was staged as T2 tumor by EUS and is an example of overstaging due to peritumorous inflammation in the deep submucosa and in the muscle layer. The hypoechoic tumor (*arrows*) infiltrates the anastomosis and adjacent parts of the stomach. On EUS, the muscularis propria cannot be delineated from the tumor (*arrowhead*), and this was interpreted as beginning invasion. *ST*, Stomach (image inverted)

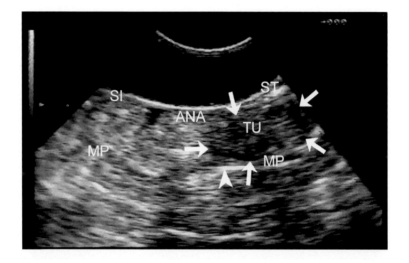

Fig. 9.14. Adenocarcinoma of the cardia in stage T3. A large hypoechoic tumor with infiltration into the distal esophagus and into the fundus is seen. The tumor is partially ulcerated with air (*arrows*) in the crater and has an irregular outer margin with tumorous pseudopodia (*arrowheads*). The investigation of the fundus is difficult, as it sometimes is a "blind" area for EUS due to the impossibility of filling this part of the stomach completely with water. Air artifacts in the ulcerated tumor can lead to incorrect T-staging.

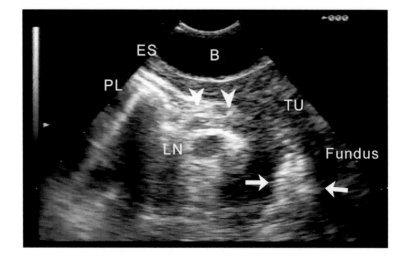

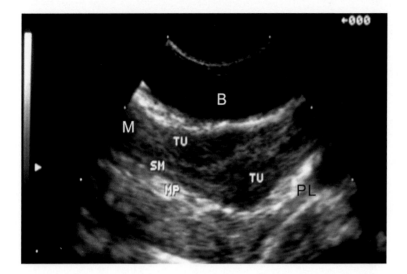

Fig. 9.15. Carcinoma of the cardia. Multifocal tumor with two hypoechoic tumor areas within the wall. The first is a superficial and polypoid part located in the mucosa; the second is deeper and partially covered by normal mucosa, but is infiltrating the submucosa and the muscularis propria. The outer margin is intact.

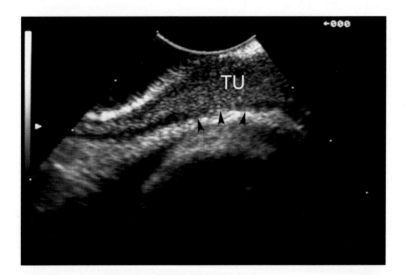

Fig. 9.16. Adenocarcinoma of the cardia in stage T2. The tumor infiltrates the distal esophagus and the cardia. The transition of the normal wall layers into the transmural hypoechoic tumor infiltration that locally includes the muscularis propria (*arrowhead*) is well demonstrated.

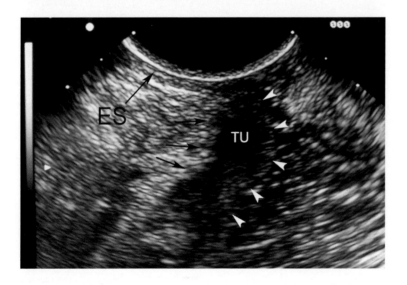

Fig. 9.17. Stage T3 carcinoma of the cardia. The cardia can be inspected from the distal esophagus (*ES*). In this case an hypoechoic cardia tumor penetrates through the wall (*arrows*). The luminal border of the tumor (*arrowheads*) is blurred by echogenic particles within the stomach.

Fig. 9.18. Linitis plastica. Circular diffuse thickening of the whole wall (1 cm) of the gastric body, with loss of the normal layer structure and thickening of all layers especially the mucosa and muscularis propria. Adjacent lymph nodes (*arrows*) are also seen. The diagnosis after resection was a stage T2N1 tumor.

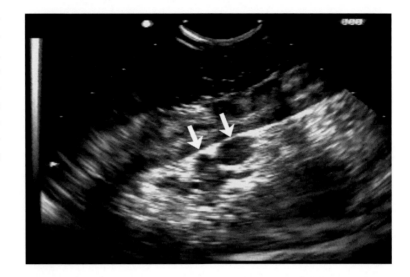

Fig. 9.19. Linitis plastica. Diffuse tumor infiltration of the antral wall with deep, hypoechoic, extended thickening predominantly of the second and the fourth layers, with preservation of the layers as distinctive structures. Typical EUS-aspect of an infiltrative growth pattern with a rigid wall are seen. The third hypoechoic "layer" on the right side is caused by ascites (*ASC*) between liver and serosa. Repeatedly negative biopsies in such cases can occur. EUS can aid in making the diagnosis via fine needle aspiration.

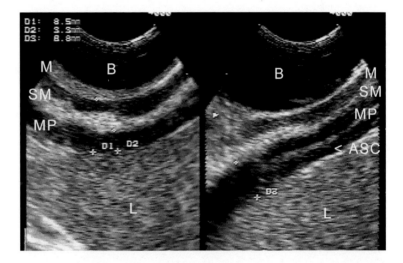

Fig. 9.20. Mucosa-associated lymphoid tissue lymphoma: A half-moon-like tumor in the antrum with a hypoechoic thickening of the mucosa and submucosa is seen. Deep hypoechoic tumor growth in the mucosa and infiltration of the submucosa are also visible. The tumor growth in this case is strictly limited to the mucosa. Gastric lymphomas can appear as polypoid lesions, as ulcerated and localized infiltrations, or as diffuse infiltration. Differentiation from other malignant tumors (carcinoma) and linitis plastica is not possible by EUS.

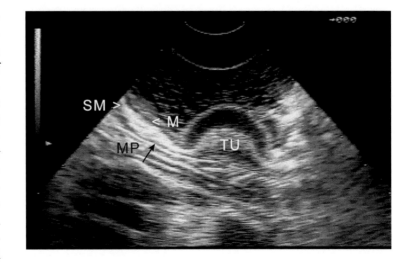

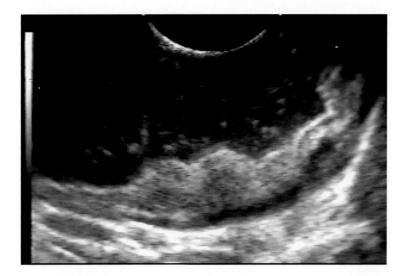

Fig. 9.21. Primary gastric lymphoma. Endosonographic image of a localized wall thickening of the mucosa, submucosa and the muscularis propria.

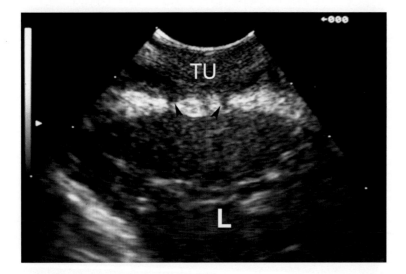

Fig. 9.22. Primary gastric lymphoma. This high-grade lymphoma of the lesser curvature penetrates the serosa (*arrowhead*), corresponding to an E-I2 lymphoma. While systemic chemotherapy is mandatory in all stages of high-grade gastric lymphoma, in low-grade gastric lymphoma, local treatment with radiotherapy and surgery is carried out in curative intent in the early stages of the disease. This must be defined by EUS. EUS is also important to evaluate remission of gastric lymphoma after eradication treatment of *Helicobacter pylori*.

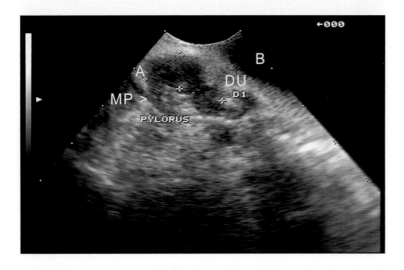

Fig. 9.23. Non-Hodgkin lymphoma. Transmural infiltration of the pylorus (++) with a hypoechoic, inhomogeneous pattern invading the proximal parts of the duodenal bulb. The balloon is partially compressed by the tumor. The interpretation of lesions in the pylorus can be very difficult due to variations in the thickness of the muscle and technical difficulties in placing the transducer correctly in the pylorus. *A,* Antrum

Fig. 9.24. *Helicobacter pylori* positive gastritis. Large gastric folds are seen with homogeneous thickening (++) involving only the inner two layers (mucosa) of the gastric wall. The water-filled gastric lumen is also seen. Especially in histologically negative cases of large gastric folds, EUS can contribute to the diagnosis prior to biopsy by excluding intramural vessels. In addition, it can define whether there is a selective thickening of only the inner layers (acute gastritis, foveolar hyperplasia, Ménétrier's disease) or of the outer layers (lymphoma, linitis).

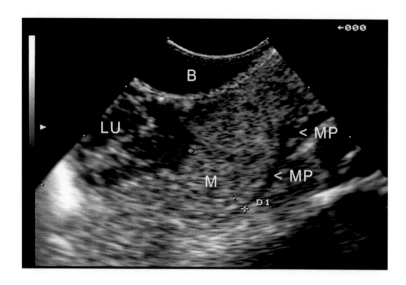

Fig. 9.25. Ménétriere's disease. The endosonographic image shows only the two inner layers (mucosa) thickened with hyperplastic gastric folds.

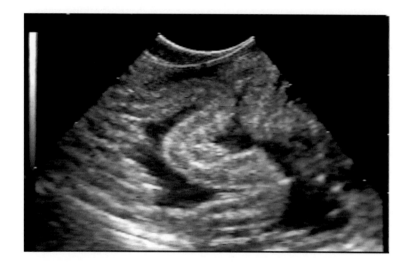

Fig. 9.26. Metastatic infiltration of the gastric wall by breast cancer. *Left* Diffuse infiltration of the wall with thickening of all wall layers in the corpus, but predominantly in the proper muscle layer (*arrowheads*). *Right* Better differentiation of the wall layers in the antrum, with ascites (*arrow*).

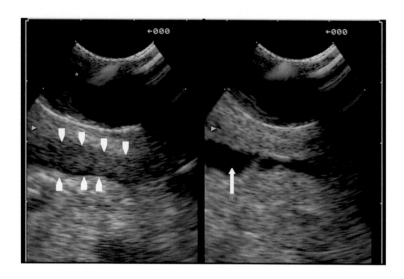

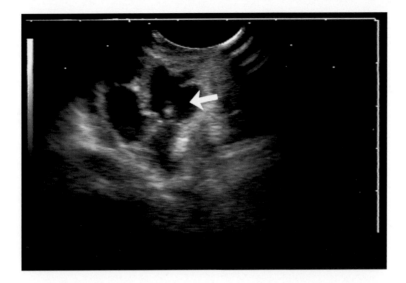

Fig. 9.27. Fundic varices. Tortuous convoluted anechoic tubular structures in the wall of the gastric fundus are seen.

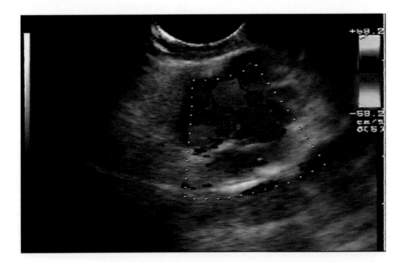

Fig. 9.28. Fundic varices. Color Doppler can easely differentiate between vascular and cystic formations in the gastric wall.

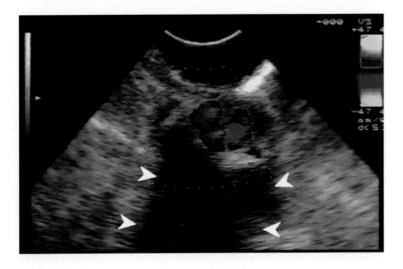

Fig. 9.29. Fundic varix. Color Doppler visualization of fundic varices with partial obliteration of one varix after therapy in a patient with portal hypertension after bleeding. The large shadow (*arrowheads*) behind the varix is caused by cyanoacrylate glue.

Fig. 9.30. Fundic varices in the submucosa (*arrow*) in B-mode (*left*) and color-mode (*right*). The submucosa is thickened because of the presence of vascular structures.

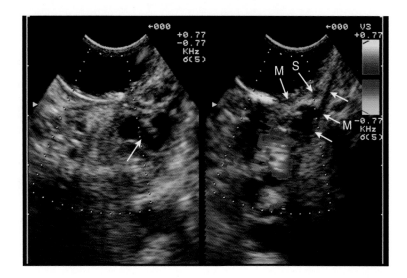

Fig. 9.31. Gastric ulcer: active, benign ulcer. Alteration of the normal layer structure with hypoechoic thickening induced by edema and inflammation and tangential artifacts from the ulcer crater (**). The crater is very well visualized due to water filling of the lumen (*LU*). EUS is unable to distinguish benign from malignant ulcers. Repeated biopsies are necessary when the diagnosis is uncertain. *Arrows*: shadow artifact.

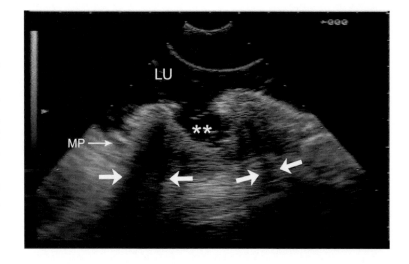

Fig. 9.32. Gastric Crohn's disease. Hypoechoic infiltration in inflammatory disease can extend beyond the serosa, mimicking a T3 cancer. In this case the transmural infiltration was caused by gastric Crohn's disease. The infiltration affects at least the subserosa (*arrowheads*). In suspected esophageal or gastric ulcers, deep and large-particle biopsies and endoscopic follow-up are necessary to confirm or exclude malignancy. EUS criteria of malignancy in suspicious ulcers only helps when clear invasion of neighboring organs is present.

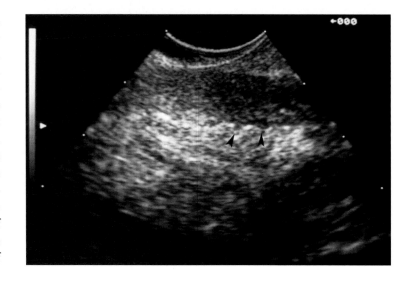

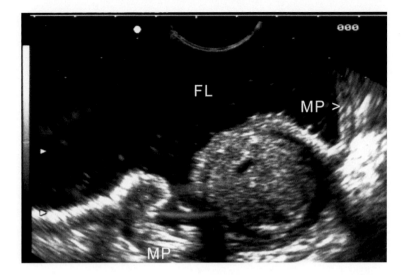

Fig. 9.33. Submucosal tumor of the stomach wall. A round and well circumscribed leiomyoma originating from the muscularis propria (*MP*) is visualized. An echo-free cystic structure is located inside the tumor. The stomach is filled with fluid (*FL*). *Arrows:* muscularis propria.

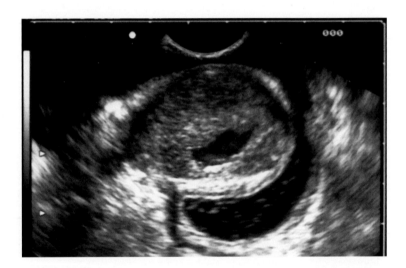

Fig. 9.34. Leiomyoma of the stomach wall. This image is taken from the same patient. A peristaltic wave has moved the position of the tumor.

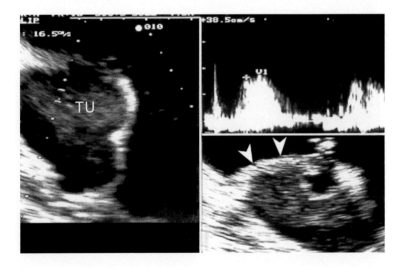

Fig. 9.35. Gastric leiomyoma. *Right*, the hypoechoic, inhomogeneous tumor shows central excavation. The tumor originates in the muscularis propria. The endoluminal part of the gastric wall is represented by the three tightly overlying anatomical layers with different echo patterns (*arrowheads*). *Left*, Tumor image (*TU*) from spectral Doppler ultrasound. *Upper right*, Correlating arterial spectrum. An ulcerated, highly vascular tumor within the gastric wall suggests the diagnosis of a leiomyoma.

Fig. 9.36. Gastric leiomyoma with borderline malignancy. The patient was admitted to the hospital with hematemesis. Endoscopy revealed a polypoid tumor with bridging folds and a central erosion, showing stigmata of bleeding. EUS demonstrates a tumor at the curvature of the stomach (*arrow*). The echo pattern of the tumor appears to be inhomogeneous with tubular structures near the tumor margins (*arrowheads*). *Left*, a normally layered gastric wall is seen.

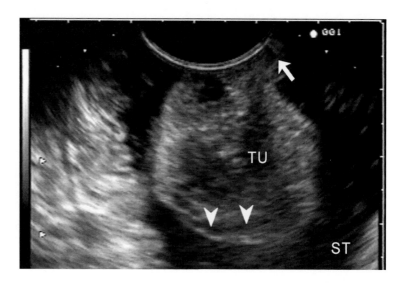

Fig. 9.37. Gastric leiomyoma (same case as in Fig. 9.36) **on color Doppler EUS.** The color Doppler mode detects large vessels (*arrows*) near the tumor margin, which is considered a pathognomonic finding of mesenchymal tumors, known to be highly vascular. However, not even color Doppler EUS can differentiate between malignant and benign mesenchymal tumors. All tumors should be resected if they are larger than 3 cm, have an inhomogeneous echo pattern, show an irregular border, or present with complications such as bleeding.

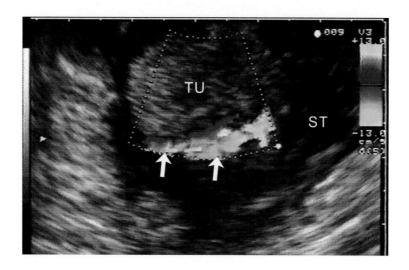

Fig. 9.38. Ganglioneurinoma. A small, well-demarcated tumor originating in the fourth layer (muscularis propria) with an inhomogeneous, hypoechoic structure. Submucosal tumors are one of the main indications for EUS in order to define the origin of the tumor. Neurogenic tumors are usually located in the submucosal layer. Leiomyomas, leiomyoblastomas, and leiomyosarcomas are located in the muscle layers. Lipomas, fibromas, or cysts are again found in the submucosa.

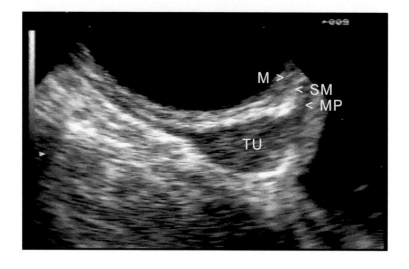

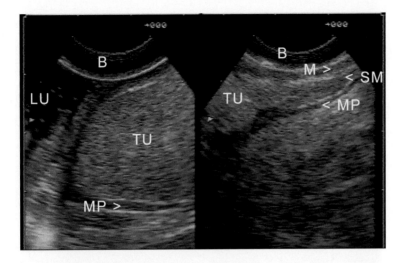

Fig. 9.39. Large lipoma in the third layer with a hyperechoic echo pattern. Lipomas are usually homogeneous, hyperechoic, well demarcated, and located in the submucosa. The hypoechoic muscularis propria can be followed underneath the lesion. *Right*, distal part of the tumor; *left*, proximal part.

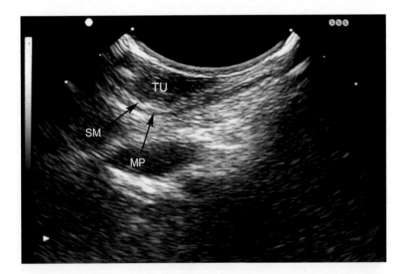

Fig. 9.40. Gastric carcinoid. This hypoechoic, strictly mucosal lesion had the typical appearance of a submucosal tumor on endoscopy, showing a smooth intact surface. Biopsy-confirmed carcinoid tissue. The tumor was completely removed endoscopically by mucosectomy.

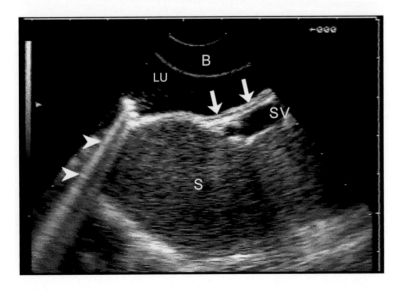

Fig. 9.41. Extraluminal compression suspected submucosal tumor in gastroscopy. The spleen is causing compression of the gastric wall. The layers of the wall can be followed over the lesion (*arrows*) and EUS clearly demonstrates the lesion to be of extraluminal origin. *Arrowheads*, air artifact; *LU*, lumen.

Fig. 9.42. Gastric polyp. Endosonographic image of a mixed reflective intraluminal mass.

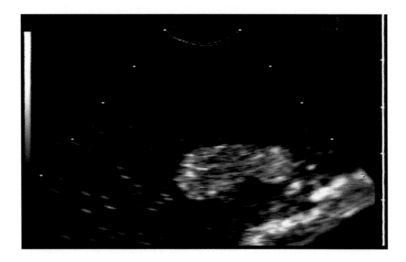

Fig. 9.43. Ascitic fluid. A small amount of echo-free fluid (*arrow*) is seen in the abdominal cavity between the stomach and the liver. *L*, Liver; *ST*, stomach wall

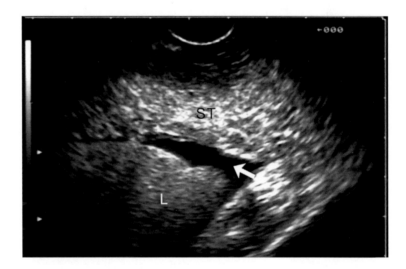

Fig. 9.44. Adenoma. A pedunculated polyp 2 cm in diameter located in the lower part of the gastric body without larger blood vessels being visible in the stalk. Histological examination after snare polypectomy showed a gastric adenoma with mild dysplasia.

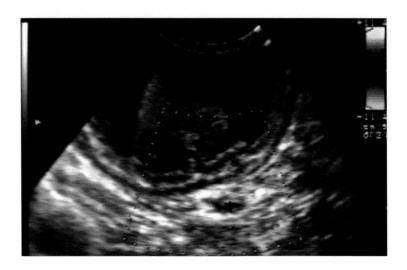

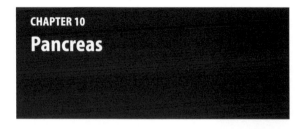

CHAPTER 10

Pancreas

E. Burmester · C. Jakobeit and L. Welp

J. Janssen and L. Greiner · P. Kann · H. Seifert

P. Vilmann · U. Will

(For abbreviations see page 175)

Fig. 10.1. Pancreatic cancer (stage T1N0). Near the confluence of the portal vein, EUS reveals a hypoechoic mass (13 mm) within the parenchyma of the head of the pancreas. The echo pattern is inhomogeneous, and the margin is irregular. The portal vein shows a hyperechoic interface echo (*arrowheads*), considered to be a major EUS criteria for ruling out tumor infiltration into the portal vein. Closer to the ultrasound transducer, all five layers of the duodenal wall are detectable (*arrow*).

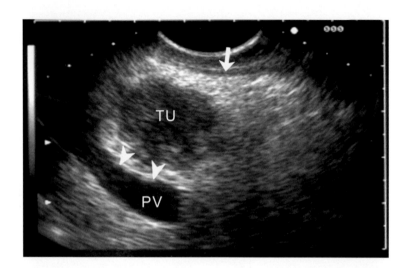

Fig. 10.2. Pancreatic cancer (stage T1N0). EUS shows a hypoechoic inhomogenous 10-mm mass with an irregular border within the parenchyma of the pancreatic tail. The splenic vein and the posterior wall of the stomach are landmarks for identifying the left pancreas. The hyperechoic line in the gastric wall is the tip of a fine needle (*arrow*), being used to perform a biopsy of the tumor mass. However, in cases of small tumors, a surgery should be seriously considered even if the fine-needle biopsy specimen reveals no cytological evidence of malignancy.

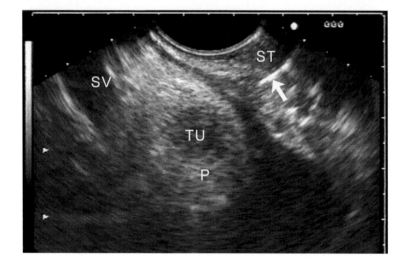

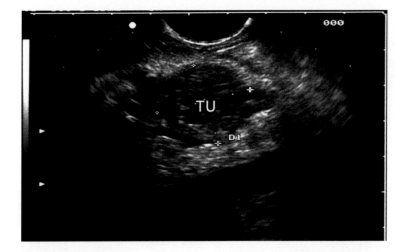

Fig. 10.3. Pancreatic cancer (stage T2). A 2.5-cm hypoechoic tumor (*TU*) is visualized, surrounded by pancreatic tissue. No invasion of adjacent structures is seen.

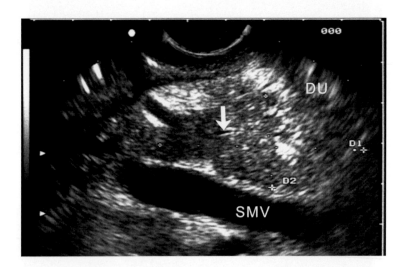

Fig. 10.4. Pancreatic cancer (stage T3). A 5.2-cm irregular tumor bordering at the superior mesenteric vein (*SMV*) is seen inside the pancreatic head. *Arrow*, pancreatic duct; *DU*, Duodenal wall

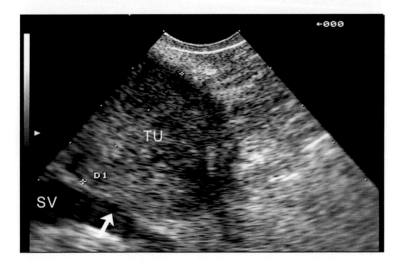

Fig. 10.5. Pancreatic cancer (stage T3). Hypoechoic tumor in the tail of the pancreas. The transducer is located in the stomach. The tumor is sharply demarcated with loss of the hyperechoic interface between tumor and the splenic vein (*SV*) (*arrow*). The loss of the tumor-vessel interface is a possible EUS sign of tumor infiltration, but false-positive findings are possible due to peritumorous inflammatory changes. The main pancreatic duct is not visible.

Fig. 10.6. Stage T4 Pancreatic cancer. This tumor is invading the dorsal gastric wall. There is focal complete transmural invasion (*arrows*) and infiltration into the muscularis propria (*arrowheads*).

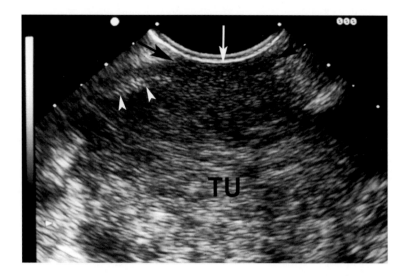

Fig. 10.7. Stage T4 pancreatic cancer. A hypoechoic lesion in the head of the pancreas is seen. The interface between the tumor and the superior mesenteric vein is lost due to tumor invasion of the vessel.

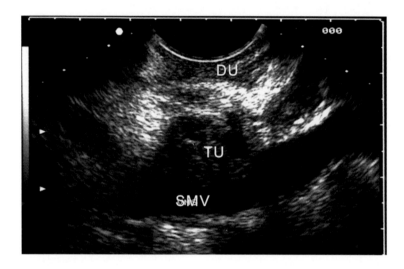

Fig. 10.8. Stage T4 carcinoma. The transducer is placed in the body of the stomach. Hypoechoic tumor infiltration of the pancreatic body with pseudopodia and infiltration of the retroperitoneal fat is seen (*arrows*). The loss of the interface between the tumor and the muscularis propria of the stomach shows the broad infiltration into the gastric wall (*arrowheads*). Vascular invasion into the splenic artery is also present.

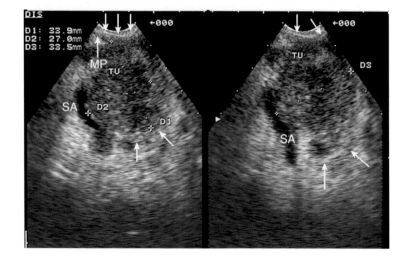

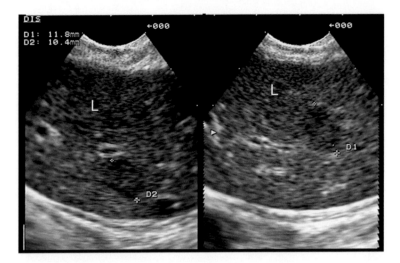

Fig. 10.9. Metastatic pancreatic cancer. Two very small hypoechoic metastases (*between the markers D1++ and D2++*) in the left liver (*L*) which were not visible on contrast-enhanced computed tomography (CT) are seen. This illustrates the necessity to attempt M staging with EUS.

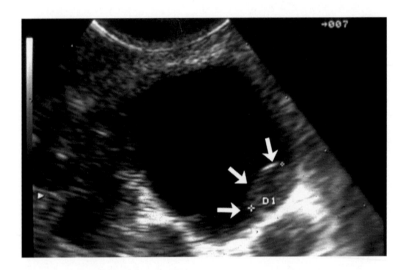

Fig. 10.10. Cystadenocarcinoma. Multicystic tumor in the pancreatic tail. The CT-guided aspirate of the cyst was cytologically negative. Note the small solid tumor in the wall of the large cyst (*arrows*), which EUS guided fine-needle aspiration demonstrated to be an adenocarcinoma. Cystic tumors of the pancreas can appear as multicystic tumors surrounded by solid tumor masses or as a single large cyst with an irregular wall and pericystic lesions. Differentiation between cystadenoma and cystadenocarcinoma is not possible by EUS imaging.

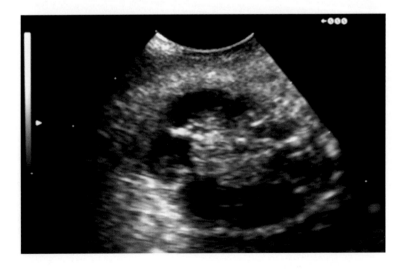

Fig. 10.11. Pancreatic cystadenoma. This rosette-like lesion within the pancreatic head is caused by a cystadenoma (histologically confirmed). The transducer is placed just below the upper duodenal curve. EUS is not able to define the histological nature of such a lesion by morphological criteria.

Fig. 10.12 a, b. Mucinous cystadenoma: a The rosette-like lesion is localized in the head of the pancreas and is caused by a cystadenoma. The tumor shows multiple large cysts which are separated by hyperechoic solid band-like structures. On power Doppler imaging, **(b)** flow signals are detected in the solid pericystic structures. This is a sign of cystic neoplasia and an indication for surgery.

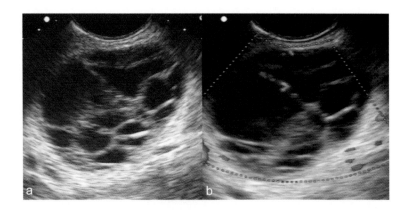

Fig. 10.13. Pancreatic metastasis of a hypernephroma. A sharply demarcated tumor (*TU*) in the body of the pancreas with a homogeneous echo pattern was identified by EUS as an endocrine tumor 6 years previously the patient had been operated on for a left renal hypernephroma. *L* = Lymph node

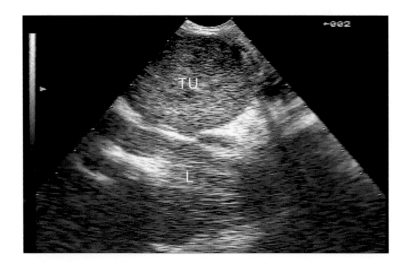

Fig. 10.14. Neuroendocrine tumor of the pancreas. A 8.7-mm hypoechoic insulinoma (*arrow*) is located in the tail of the pancreas. *SV*, Splenic vein; *REV*, left renal vein

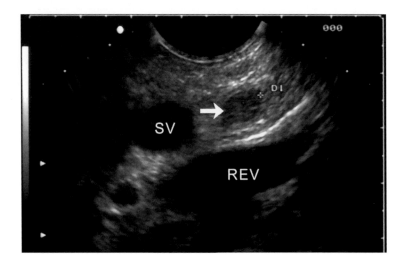

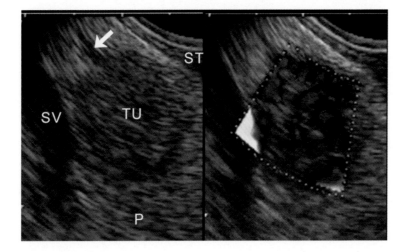

Fig. 10.15. Insulinoma. The tumor, scanned from the gastric fundus, is located within the pancreatic parenchyma. Left, a hypoechoic signal pattern of the tumor near the pancreatic duct (*arrow*) is seen. The splenic vein and the posterior wall of the stomach are normal. After intravenous administration of an ultrasound contrast medium (Levovist), various echo signals are found in the tumor, which correspond to vessels. As with other neuroendocrine tumors, insulinomas are highly vascularized.

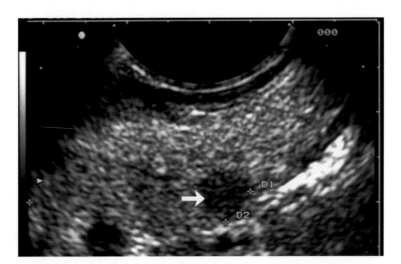

Fig. 10.16. Neuroendocrine tumor of the pancreas. A 6.6-mm gastrinoma (*arrows*) is seen in the pancreatic parenchyma. The transducer is located in the stomach, compressing the stomach wall layers against the body of the pancreas.

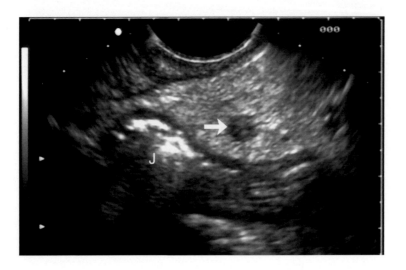

Fig. 10.17. Neuroendocrine tumor of the pancreas. A 10-mm hypoechoic carcinoid tumor (*arrows*) is seen in the pancreatic body. The transducer is placed against the gastric wall. The small intestine is seen with reflections caused by intraluminal air.

Fig. 10.18. Neuroendocrine tumor of the pancreas. A 2.5 cm hypoechoic carcinoid tumor adjacent to the pancreas is located between the celiac axis and the superior mesenteric artery. The aorta is seen in the longitudinal plane.

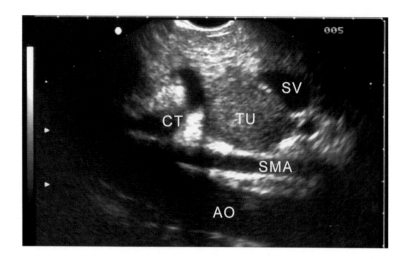

Fig. 10.19. Somatostatinoma of the pancreatic head. The tumor mass (approx. 2 cm) shows a hypoechoic, inhomogeneous pattern and infiltrates the duodenal wall. In and around the tumor, multiple tubular structures are visible (*arrowheads*). The EUS diagnosis of vascular structures (with the help of Doppler EUS) makes a neuroendocrine tumor more likely. In contrast, ductal adenocarcinomas of the pancreas are usually poorly vascularized.

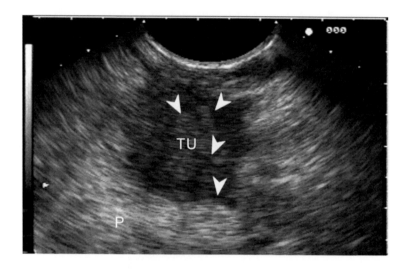

Fig. 10.20. Somatostatinoma (same patient as in Fig. 10.19), visualized by color power Doppler imaging. Prior to ultrasound scanning, contrast medium (Levovist) is administered intravenously. EUS using color power Doppler mode shows multiple vessels in the tumor located in the head of the pancreas (*arrowheads*). This finding is correlated with a tubular, hypoechoic signal pattern on the B-mode EUS and suggests a neuroendocrine pancreatic tumor. The gastroduodenal artery (*arrow*) is located tangentially to the tumor.

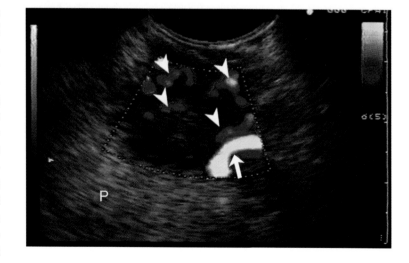

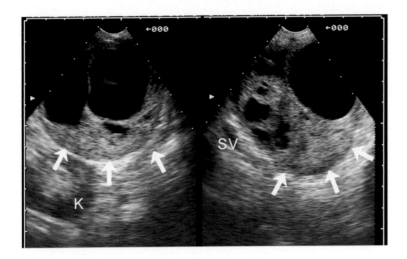

Fig. 10.21. Malignant endocrine tumor (histologically unclassified). A large sharply demarcated tumor (*arrows*) with a hypoechoic capsule, solid tissue, and multiple cysts is seen. *SV*: Compressed splenic vein. Endocrine tumors usually present as hypoechoic homogeneous, well-demarcated lesions; rarely, hyperechoic tumors with cystic areas and calcifications can be observed.

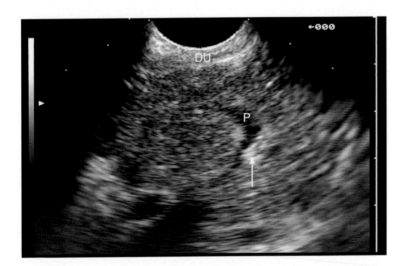

Fig. 10.22. Chronic pancreatitis (early form) in the head of the pancreas with hyperechoic parenchymal changes (*arrow*) due to fibrosis. The pancreatic duct has irregular walls and shows evidence of moderate stenosis. The transducer is located in the duodenum.

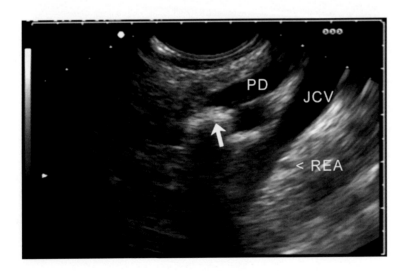

Fig. 10.23. Stone in the pancreatic duct seen on longitudinal scanning from the distal duodenum. Within the uncinate process of the pancreas, a dilated pancreatic duct containing a hyperechoic stone (*arrow*) with acoustic shadowing is detectable. Behind the pancreas, the inferior vena cava and the right renal artery are visible. EUS is the appropriate method to further specify a pancreatic duct structure or obstruction on ERCP.

Fig. 10.24. Chronic pancreatitis. Typical ductal changes in moderate chronic pancreatitis of the main duct are seen. These changes include pancreatic duct dilation, an irregular pancreatic duct border, partially increased wall echoes, and an inhomogeneous, focal hyperechoic parenchymal pattern due to fibrosis and small calcifications.

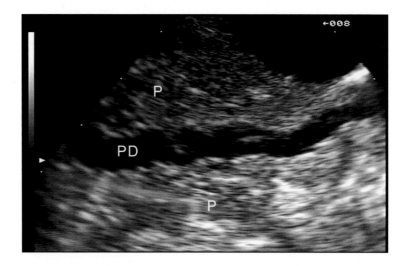

Fig. 10.25. Severe chronic pancreatitis (*arrowheads*). Advanced chronic pancreatitis with calcifications in the head of the pancreas, irregular duct borders with dilation of the distal duct, and a long stenotic segment are seen (*small arrows*). An intraductal stone is visualized (*arrow*) as well as is atrophic parenchyma in the body. EUS is not superior to ERCP in detection of duct obstructions, but can contribute in identifiying the etiology of the obstruction (tumor, stone, etc.) if ERCP cannot demonstrate the distal parts of the duct beyond a stenosis. The transducer is located in the duodenum.

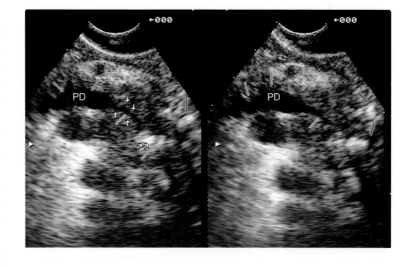

Fig. 10.26. Chronic pancreatitis with calcifications. A longitudinal EUS section through the distal body of the pancreas reveals multiple hyperechoic foci with postacoustic shadowing in the pancreatic parenchyma (*arrows*). The superior mesenteric vein behind the body of the pancreas shows no irregularities. EUS examination of the pancreas and the neighboring vessels can be difficult because of ultrasound-related artifacts and the enlarged organ. As a result, small carcinomas are difficult to identify in an inflamed organ.

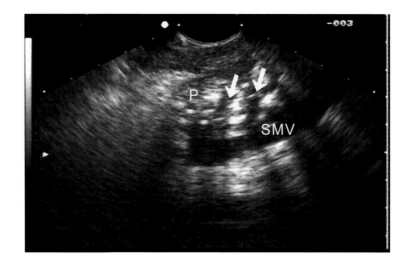

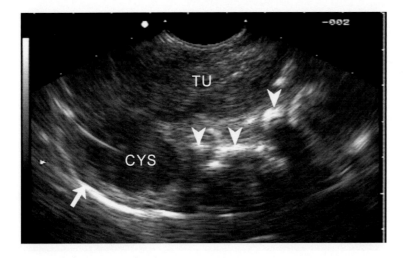

Fig. 10.27. Chronic inflammatory pseudotumor. This is a longitudinal EUS section from the proximal duodenum. The pancreas is enlarged and reveals an inhomogeneous echo pattern. The lumen of the descending duodenum (*arrow*) is narrowed by a chronic pseudocyst (*Cys*). The shadows indicate calcifications of the parenchyma (*arrowheads*). Close to the EUS transducer, the head of the pancreas reveals a different, more hypoechoic pattern. This suggests the presence of carcinoma. EUS guided fine-needle puncture is recommended in these situations.

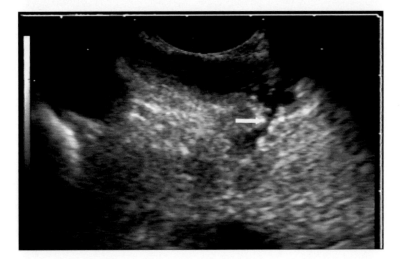

Fig. 10.28. Inflammatory stenosis of the papilla of Vater. After papillotomy, a hypoechoic tumorous lesion in the peripapillary region is seen. This is why EUS may be indicated before ERCP to diagnose the cause of jaundice (*arrow* pancreatic duct).

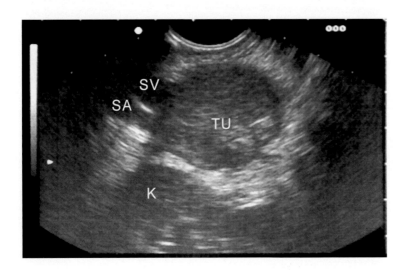

Fig. 10.29. Focal pancreatitis in the pancreatic tail. The pancreatic tail is enlarged, with smooth margins around a mass. The EUS signal pattern of the mass is hypoechoic and relatively homogeneous. As the nature of this finding cannot be clarified by EUS alone, EUS guided fine-needle biopsy was subsequently performed. Histological analysis showed an infiltration of pancreatic tissue with predominantly lymphocytes and plasma cells, which in combination with the clinical findings suggested the diagnosis of an inflammatory mass. After 6 weeks of follow-up, the swelling was no longer detectable.

Fig. 10.30. Pseudocyst in the pancreatic tail. A typical cyst is demonstrated, with the splenic artery, the left adrenal gland, and the left kidney being visible. All layers of the wall of the gastric fundus are clearly distinguishable. Such pseudocysts, which are mostly the sequelae of pancreatitis, should not be approached by EUS guided fine needle puncture (because of the increased risk of infection) if there are no signs of a tumorous cystic structure or thickened cyst wall.

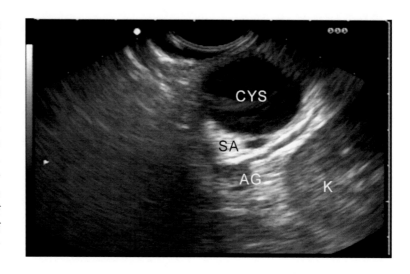

Fig. 10.31. Infradiaphragmatic pancreatic pseudocyst in the pancreatic tail region (*right*) and supradiaphragmatic pancreatogenic intrapleural fluid collection (*left*) with adjacent pulmonary air (*left below*). The transducer is in the lower esophagus or cardia and is directed in the left-posterior direction. Both cystic lesions are organized, as each has a fibrous wall.

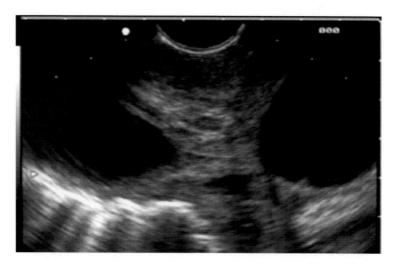

Fig. 10.32. Pancreatic pseudocyst. A small "tumorlike" pancreatic pseudocyst (++), 12 weeks after a severe attack of acute pancreatitis, is located in the bursa behind the gastric wall (*GW*). Hypoechoic necrosis near the cyst (*arrows*) and a solid interval echo pattern caused by necrotic material are seen. EUS guided puncture only showed sterile material. Differentiation between a tumor and a pseudocyst is impossible in this situation.

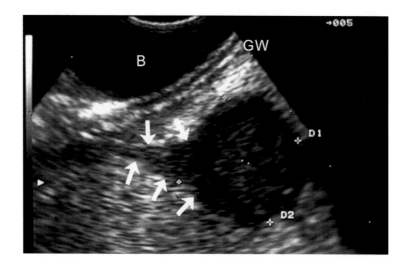

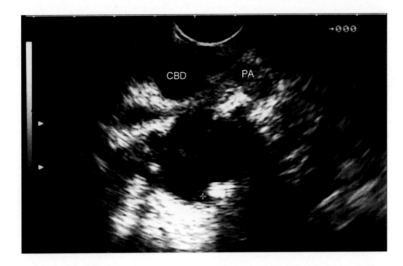

Fig. 10.33. Pancreatic pseudocyst. The transducer is located in the second part of the duodenum and held against the papilla (*PA*). The common bile duct (*CBD*) is located immediately below the transducer. Below the CBD, a pseudocyst is seen in the pancreatic head with a diameter of 19 mm. Note the attenuation of the ultrasound beam behind the cyst.

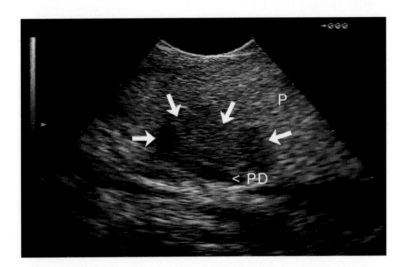

Fig. 10.34. Acute focal pancreatitis. This image is from a young patient with a small irregular hypoechoic lesion near the pancreatic duct. This lesion was identified 6 weeks after an episode of focal acute pancreatitis. Note the "tumor-like" aspect of the lesion. EUS is unable to differentiate these inflammatory changes from malignant lesions.

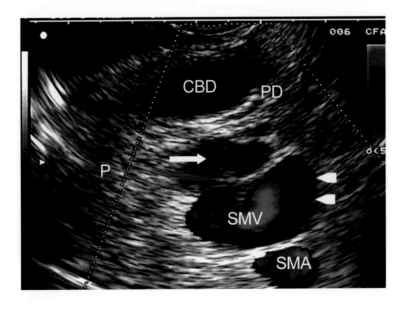

Fig. 10.35. Focal acute pancreatitis with a thrombotic complication: In the pancreas, a focal hypoechoic irregular structure near the superior mesenteric vein is seen (*arrow*). The pancreatic duct and common bile duct are normal. In the superior mesenteric vein, an inhomogenous color Doppler signal without flow signals is seen near the wall of the vein (*arrowheads*). This suggests a thrombus adherent to the wall.

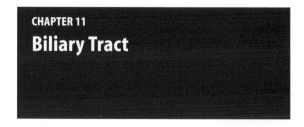

CHAPTER 11

Biliary Tract

E. Burmester · C. Jakobeit and L.Welp

J. Janssen and L. Greiner · P. Vilmann · U. Will

(For abbreviations see page 175)

Fig. 11.1. Choledocholithiasis. A gallstone (*GS*) 5 mm in diameter is seen in the distal common bile duct (*CBD*). The transducer is positioned against the papillary region in the second part of the duodenum.

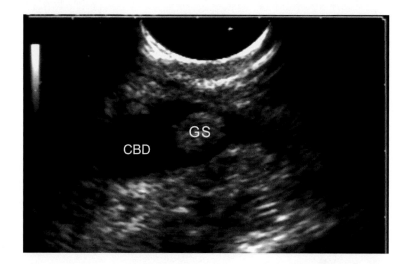

Fig. 11.2. Choledocholithiasis. A small choledochal stone in the distal part of the common bile duct showing as hyperechoic foci (*arrows*) with acoustic shadowing (*arrowheads*) behind the stone in a patient with a negative ERCP. EUS has a high accuracy, comparable to that of ERCP, in detecting choledocholithiasis. However, it does not offer the possibility of stone removal. *LU*, Water-filled duodenal lumen; *PAP*, Papilla

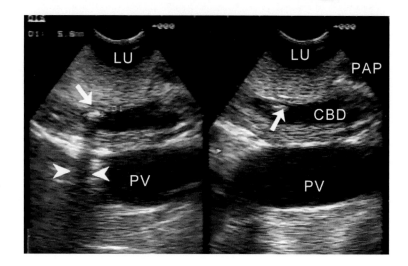

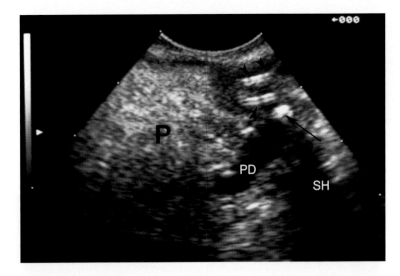

Fig. 11.3. Bile duct stone impacted in the ampulla. After sphincterotomy and extraction of bile duct stones, this patient suffered from recurrent episodes of pancreatitis. ERCP suggested an inflammatory ampullary stenosis without showing any biliary or pancreatic stones. A biliary drainage catheter (*arrowheads*) was inserted. Finally, EUS confirmed an occluding stone within the ampulla of the pancreatic duct (*arrows*). This stone was possibly displaced from the common bile duct. After removing the stone, the patient recovered completely.

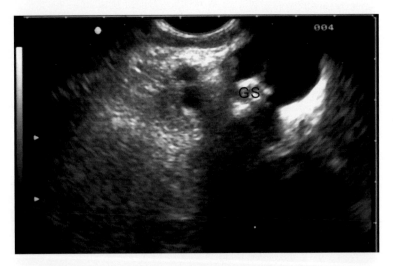

Fig. 11.4. Choledocholithiasis. A gallstone (*GS*) located in the middle part of the common bile duct is visualized from the first part of the duodenum. The CBD is therefore seen in a transverse section. Note the acoustic shadow created behind the echogenic stone.

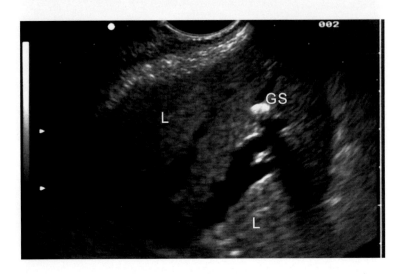

Fig. 11.5. Intrahepatic cholelithiasis. A gallstone (*GS*) is seen in an intrahepatic bile duct. Note the shadow created behind the hyperechoic stone. (*L*) Liver

Fig. 11.6. Gallbladder polyp. A small, hyperechoic polyp, (*arrow*) 5 mm in diameter, is seen in the gallbladder lumen (*GB*). The transducer is located in the first part of the duodenum.

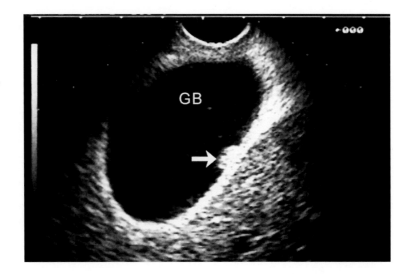

Fig. 11.7. Small polyp *(arrow)* **at the wall of the gallbladder without** any signs of infiltration. This tumor was found by chance and was not confirmed histologically. No definitive diagnostic EUS-criteria exist to describe the nature of the polyp. As it may be an adenoma, follow-up is necessary. The transducer is located in the duodenal bulb and pulled back against the pylorus (*arrowhead*).

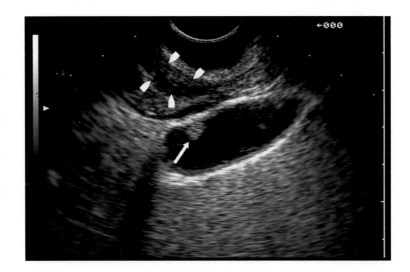

Fig. 11.8. Gallbladder carcinoma. An endosonographic picture of a large polypoid gallbladder carcinoma in the corpus.

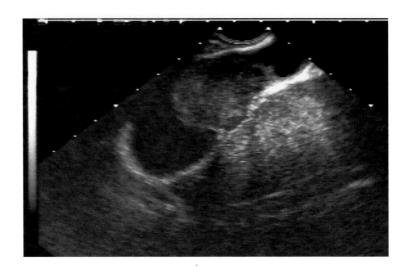

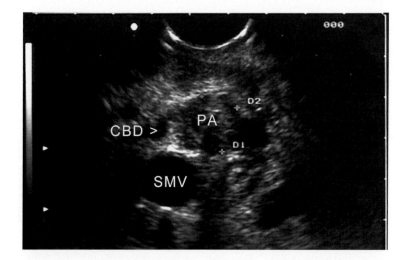

Fig. 11.9. Intrapapillary carcinoma. The transducer is located in the second part of the duodenum. A hypoechoic tumor is visualized in the intrapapillary part of the CBD. Invasion of the surrounding structures can also be seen. *CBD*, Common bile duct; *PA*, papilla of Vater; *SMV*, superior mesenteric vein.

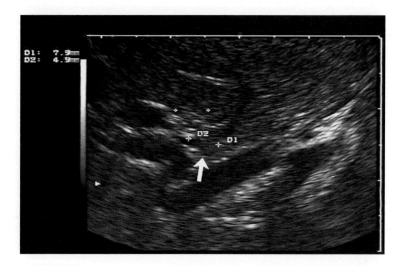

Fig. 11.10. Klatskin tumor. This endosonographic image shows a hypoechoic tumor mass in the region of the hepatic hilum obstructing the bifurcation.

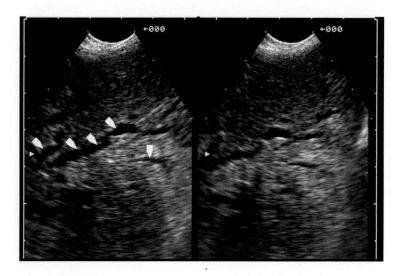

Fig. 11.11. Klatskin Tumor: This section through the left lobe of the liver demonstrates dilated intrahepatic ducts (*arrowheads*) with a hyperechoic pattern of the parenchyma that is interpreted as infiltration. The diagnosis was confirmed by ERCP, MRI and laparoscopy.

CHAPTER 12
Papilla of Vater

E. Burmester · C. Jakobeit

P. Vilmann · U. Will

(For abbreviations see page 175)

Fig. 12.1. Adenoma of the papilla of Vater. This adenoma of the papilla is covered by duodenal folds (*arrows*). Water instillation into the duodenum and/or balloon insufflation improves the ultrasound visualization. The adenoma of the papilla, growing within the duodenal mucosa, shows a homogeneous, hypoechoic signal pattern. The submucosa (*arrowheads*) and the muscularis propria have a normal thickness without evidence of infiltration. *Left*, an oblique scanning artifact can be seen. The broadened muscularis propria (*grey arrow*) should also be noted.

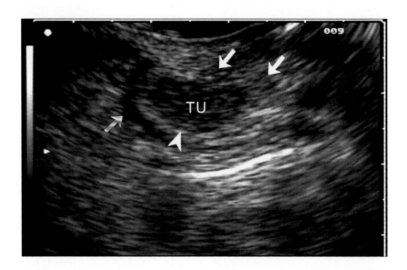

Fig. 12.2. Adenoma of the papilla of Vater. The papilla shows a homogeneous, hyperechoic signal pattern and appears to be enlarged while the pancreatic duct has a normal caliber. No enlarged lymph nodes are detectable, and the muscularis propria of the duodenal wall is clearly demonstrated (*arrow*). These EUS-based criteria are of great importance in deciding on treatment options. For example, they aid in determining whether endoscopic resection of an adenoma of the papilla is possible. However, EUS cannot differentiate between adenomas and early carcinomas.

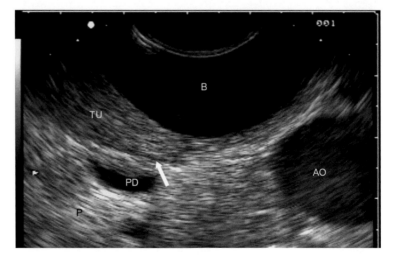

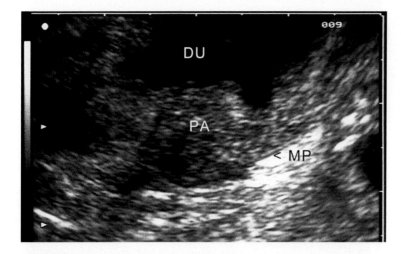

Fig. 12.3. Tumor of the papilla of Vater. Polypoid tissue of the papilla can be seen. The lumen of the duodenum (*DU*) is filled with water. The muscularis propria (*MP*) is intact underneath the polyp. The tumor was histopathologically verified as an adenoma with dysplasia.

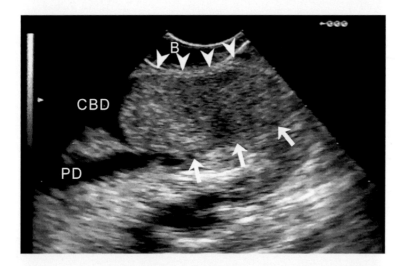

Fig. 12.4. Stage T1 adenocarcinoma of the papilla. A large, oval tumor of the papilla (*arrows*) with extrahepatic cholestasis and preservation of the duodenal wall layers is seen (*arrowheads*). The dilated common bile duct and main pancreatic duct are visualized. The tumor is soft and partially compressed by the balloon. Note that it is impossible to differentiate between an adenoma, dysplasia, and T1 carcinoma by EUS imaging alone.

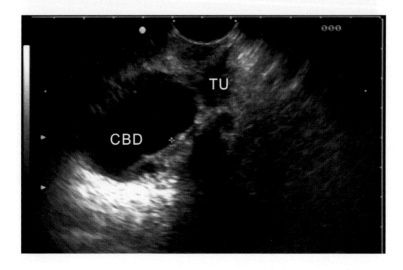

Fig. 12.5. Carcinoma of the papilla of Vater. A hypoechoic tumor is outlined by the papilla of Vater. The common bile duct is dilated (2.1 cm).

Fig. 12.6. Stage T2 carcinoma of the papilla of Vater. A hypoechoic tumor is seen in the region of the papilla of Vater (maximum diameter is 2.0 cm).

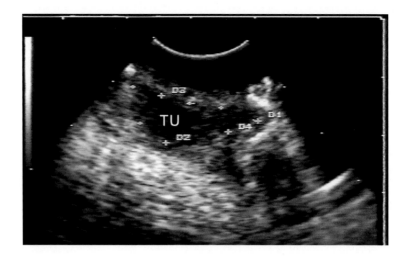

Fig. 12.7. Stage T3N1 carcinoma of the papilla of Vater. In the peripapillary region around the dilated pancreatic duct, there is a hypoechoic mass with irregular margins. This suggests a carcinoma of the papilla of Vater. A stent was inserted (*arrow*) into the common bile duct to treat the obstructive jaundice. Attached to the tumor, a small 5-mm lymph node was detectable (*arrowhead*). In the majority of cases, the type of masses in the pre-ampullary area cannot be classified by EUS alone.

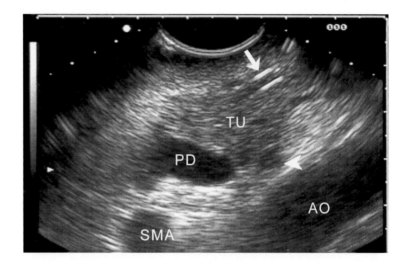

Fig. 12.8. Papillitis. This "pseudotumor" shows a hypoechoic, inhomogeneous signal pattern with an irregular contour in the ampulla of Vater. The pancreatic duct (*arrow*) has a normal caliber. Inflammatory and malignant lesions of the ampulla of Vater cannot be distinguished by EUS. The finding demonstrated here requires sphincterotomy and a deep biopsy to rule out a malignant tumor within the ampulla of Vater.

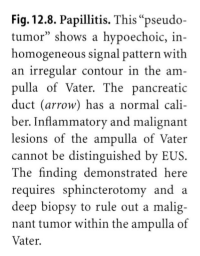

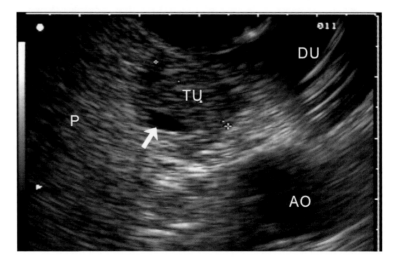

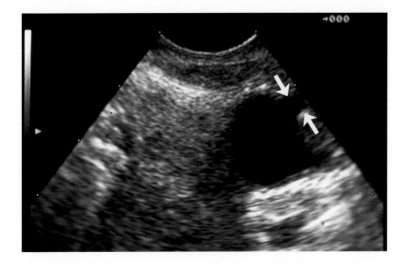

Fig. 12.9. Duodenal diverticulum. A water-filled, small periampullary diverticulum is seen in the duodenum (*arrows*, diverticulum neck). Diverticula can cause artifacts and lead to misinterpretation of a mass lesion.

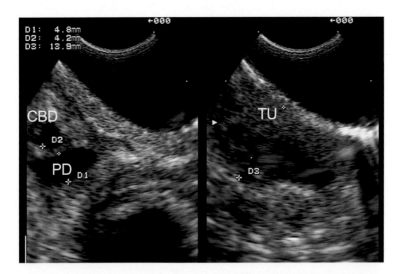

Fig. 12.10. Non-functional endocrine tumor (somatostatinoma) *Right:* A tumor in the duodenal wall (D3) is seen that is located slightly proximal to the papilla. Destruction of all wall layers is present. *Left:* The prepapillary region is not infiltrated by the tumor. The common bile duct and the pancratic duct are not dilated.

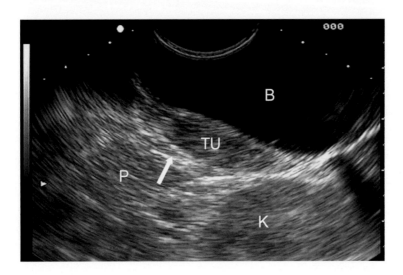

Fig. 12.11. Carcinoid tumor of the papilla of Vater: The papilla of Vater is enlarged. The tumor shows a hypoechoic structure, but the muscularis propria (*arrow*) and the pancreas are regular without signs of infiltration. There are no locoregional lymph nodes. The tumor was endoscopically radically resected. The patient has since then been tumor-free (follow-up 1 year).

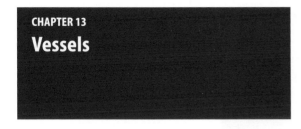

CHAPTER 13
Vessels

E. Burmester · C. Jakobeit and L. Welp

P. Vilmann · U. Will · M. Wittenberg

(For abbreviations see page 175)

Fig. 13.1. Stenosis of the celiac axis. Color Doppler examination demonstrates turbulence due to a stenosis of the celiac axis. The transducer is located in the stomach. The aorta is seen in longitudinal section.

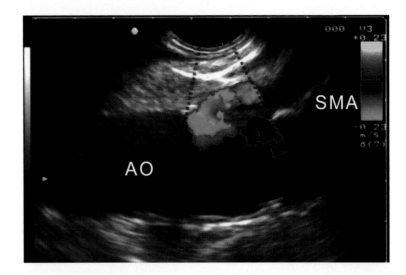

Fig. 13.2. Advanced lung cancer (SCLC) with invasion into the right pulmonary artery (RPA). EUS reveals a large inhomogenous, predominantly hypoechoic tumor which infiltrates the arterial wall over about one third of the circumference. The transverse contour of the *RPA* is markedly deformed. There is no demarcation between the anechoic lumen and the margin of the tumor. The *arrows* show the sharp borders of the invasive tumor.

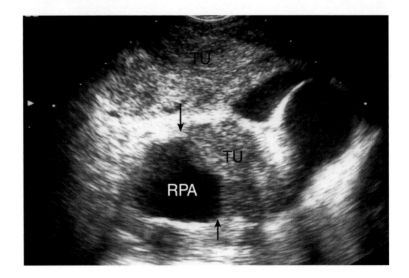

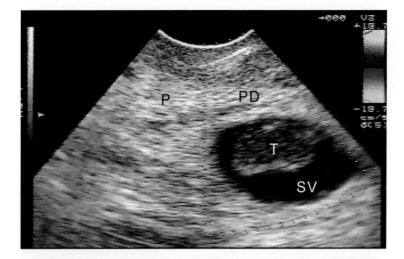

Fig. 13.3. Thrombus (*T*) of unknown etiology in the splenic vein at the confluence. The thrombus is floating in the lumen and is surrounded by blood. The thrombus is adherent to the wall of the vessel.

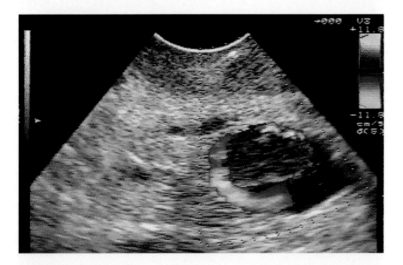

Fig. 13.4. Thrombus. The same case as above with color Doppler visualization of the thrombus in the splenic vein and typical portal venous flow.

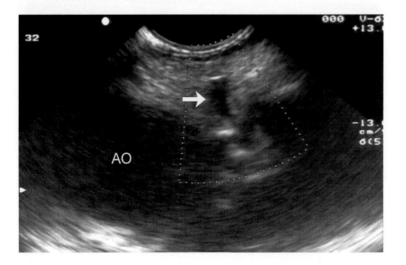

Fig. 13.5. Aberrant arterial vessel (*arrow*) in the subaortic region ("aortopulmonary window"). Hypoechoic oval lesions normally represent lymph nodes, but atypical arteries can imitate such findings (see Fig. 13.6).

Fig. 13.6. Same case as in Fig. 13.5. The Doppler technique reveals clearly that the hypoechoic oval lesion is not a lymph node but an aberrant artery. This underlines the necessity of a careful examination, especially before performing puncture.

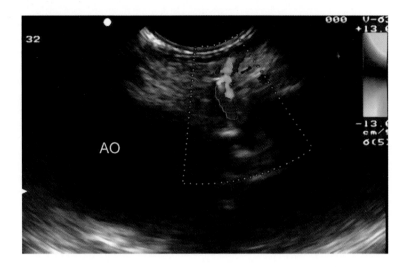

Fig. 13.7. Hemangioma of the stomach wall. A submucosal hemangioma of the stomach wall in a patient with Osler-Webber-Rendu disease. The stomach is filled with water. Only a submucosal swelling can be seen (see Fig. 13.8).

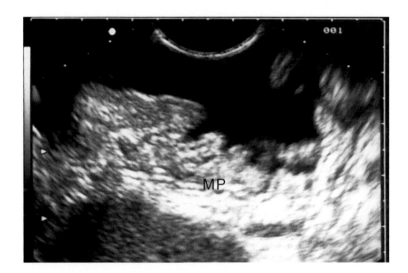

Fig. 13.8. Hemangioma of the stomach wall (same case as in Fig. 13.7). This is the corresponding image using power Doppler examination. Flow is clearly outlined due to a 1.5 cm submucosal hemangioma.

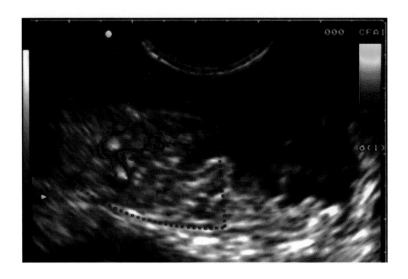

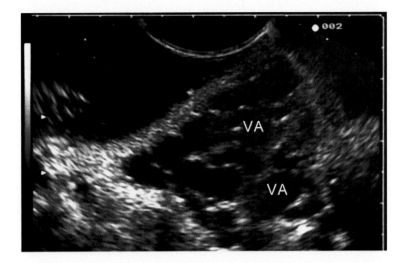

Fig. 13.9. Duodenal varices. Multiple varices are seen (*VA*) in the submucosa of the duodenal wall. Small septae separate the hypoechoic lumen of the varices (see Fig. 13.10).

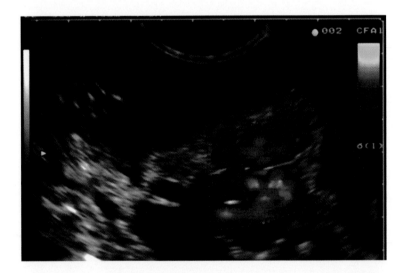

Fig. 13.10. Duodenal varices. The corresponding image to Figure 13.9 using power Doppler examination. Flow is clearly outlined in the intraduodenal varices.

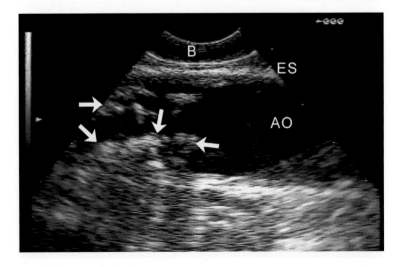

Fig. 13.11. Aortic calcifications. Calcifications (*arrows*) at the irregular aortic wall with typical hyperechoic round confluent echoes and acoustic shadowing. A normal-appearing esophagus and a longitudinal scan of part III of the aorta are seen.

Fig. 13.12. Cavernous transformation of the portal vein. This is an endosonographic image of large peripancreatic vessels in a patient with cavernomatous portal vein transformation.

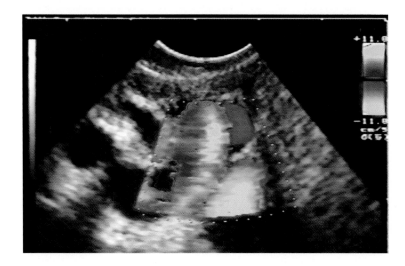

Fig. 13.13. Arteria lienalis aneurysm after severe pancreatitis. On trans-abdominal ultrasound, the semi-cystic lesion was interpretated as a pancreatic pseudocyst. *Left:* EUS demonstrated a round, onion-skin like tumor (*arrows*) with an eccentric, cystic lesion. *Right:* EUS color Doppler showed arterial signals in the cystic part and diagnosed a A. lienalis aneurysm. The diagnosis was confirmed at surgery.

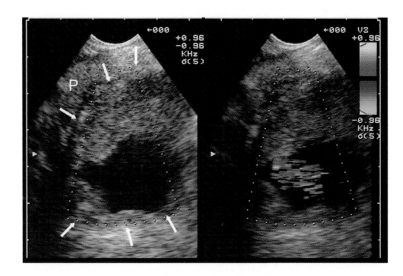

Fig. 13.14. Aortic aneurysm: The transducer is located in the second portion of the duodenum and shows a lateral section through the aorta. The vessel is dilated with partial thrombosis of the lumen. The color Doppler shows flow in the free lumen.

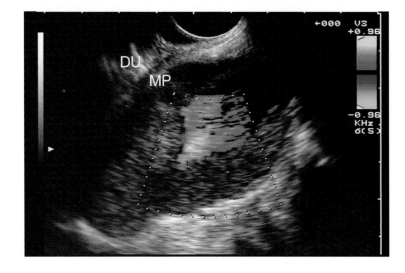

CHAPTER 14
Adrenal Glands

J.-U. Erk · P. Kann
U. Will · M. Wittenberg

(For abbreviations see page 175)

Fig. 14.1. Small adenoma of the left adrenal cortex (ACA Conn's adenoma). The diagnosis was confirmed by histological examination.

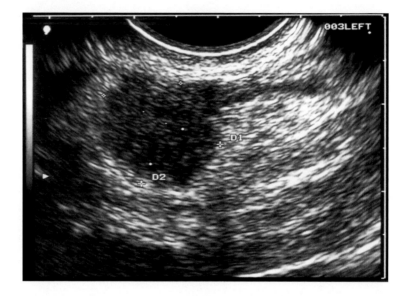

Fig. 14.2. Nodular hyperplasia of the left adrenal gland in ACTH-independent Cushing's syndrome. The diagnosis was confirmed by histological examination.

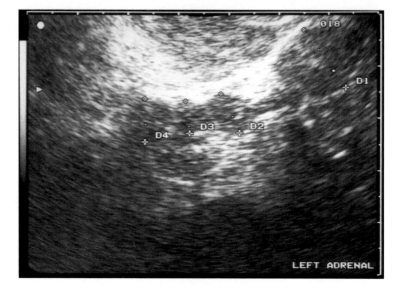

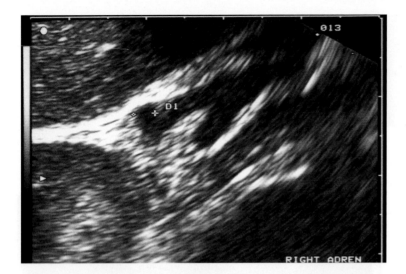

Fig. 14.3. A small nodule of the right adrenal cortex in late onset adrenogenital syndrome (heterozygous 21-hydroxylase-deficiency).

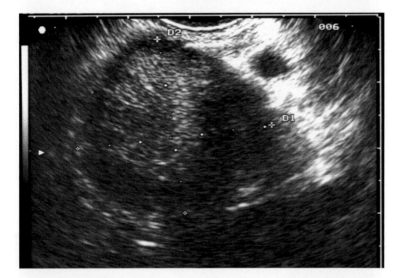

Fig. 14.4. A large nonfunctional adenoma of the left adrenal cortex. The diagnosis was confirmed by histological examination.

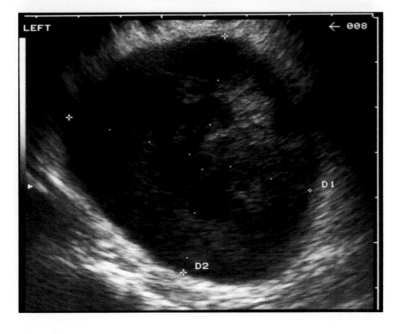

Fig. 14.5. A malignant B-cell-lymphoma of the left adrenal gland (diagnosis confirmed by FNA).

Fig. 14.6. Pheochromocytoma. A homogeneous, sharply demarcated hyperechoic tumor of the left adrenal gland region is seen. Specific histologic diagnoses (as shown in Fig. 14.4–14.7) cannot be provided by EVS imaging alone.

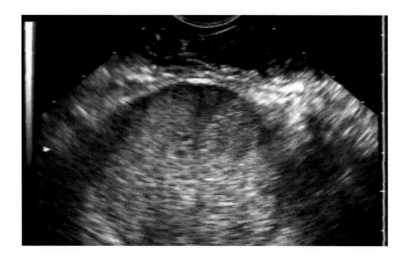

Fig. 14.7. Typical endosonographic features of a metastasis in the adrenal gland (*left*), showing an oval mass (diameter 37 mm) with sharp borders and an inhomogenous, hyperechoic echostructure. *Line*: the preserved remainder of the gland.

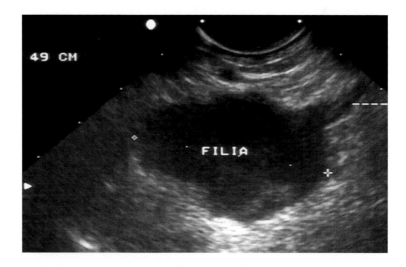

Fig. 14.8. Cyst of the left adrenal gland (D, 4.9 cm). An oval, nearly anechoic lesion with dorsal amplification of the echo reflexes. Internal hyperechoic foci can be taken as a sign for various compartments and partially solid tissue. This pattern was not detected by computed tomography (CT) or by magnetic resonance imaging (MRI). The association of the cyst with the adrenal gland was confirmed by EUS and by CT and MRI.

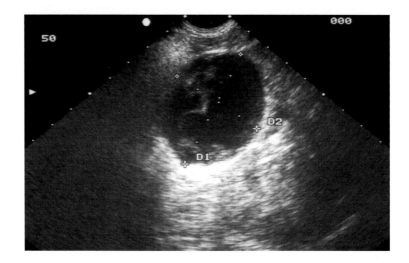

CHAPTER 15

Miscellaneous Findings

C. Jakobeit and L. Welp · J. Janssen · L. Greiner
P. Vilmann · U. Will · M. Wittenberg

(For abbreviations see page 175)

Fig. 15.1. Hemangioma of the liver. *Outlined:* Two small, hyperechoic hemangiomas of the liver (L). The transducer is placed against the stomach wall. The diaphragm is also seen (lower left).

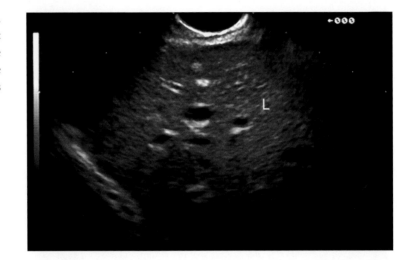

Fig. 15.2. Hemangioma of the left lobe of the liver (L). This small hyperechoic lesion of the left liver is without a hypoechoic halo (*arrowhead*) and was seen by chance on EUS. The echo pattern is typical for a hemangioma and no further diagnostic workup is needed.

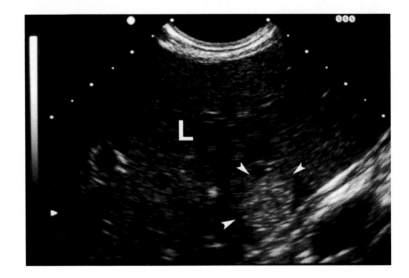

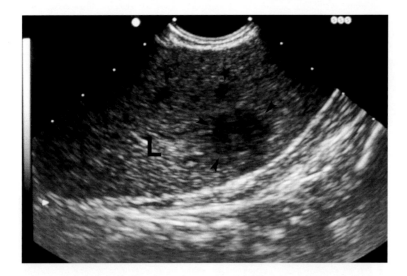

Fig. 15.3. Liver metastases. EUS is able to detect very small focal lesions in the left lobe and parts of the right lobe of the liver. In this patient with pancreatic cancer, there are some small metastases in the left lobe of the liver that measure between 2 and 11 mm in size (*arrows*). It is recommended to use EUS to examine at least the left lobe of the liver in patients with known neoplastic disease.

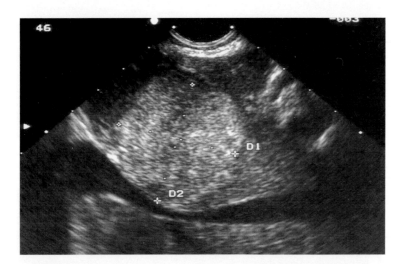

Fig. 15.4. Metastasis to the liver with compression of the inferior vena cava. A round, hyperechoic metastasis with a slight, but clear, hypoechoic margin, inhomogeneous internal echoes, and compression of the inferior vena cava is seen. The tumor margin at the IVC is sharply delineated, and thus, there is no evidence of infiltration.

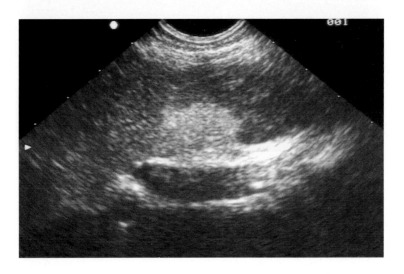

Fig. 15.5. Fatty infiltration of the liver. Echogenic lesions of the liver are ambiguous. A focal echodense pattern in the liver is compatible with fatty infiltration. The echoes in this lesion are uniform. The natural course of the vessels is preserved and the margins are sharp without a halo. Differentiation from a hemangioma is sometimes difficult. In this case, computed tomography revealed the diagnosis.

Fig. 15.6. Duplication cyst of the esophagus. A cystic lesion is detected in the distal third of the esophagus. The cyst narrows the lumen of the esophagus and the inferior vena cava (*ICV*). Although it is certain that the cyst is located in the esophageal wall, the exact layer cannot be identified. The finding is an indication for endoscopic cystotomy with a diathermy needle knife. The definitive diagnosis is then made by biopsy.

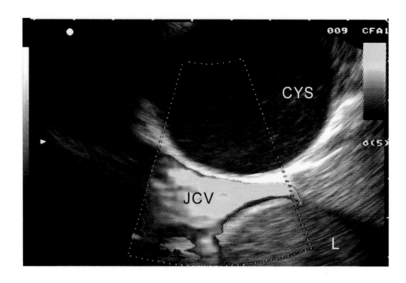

Fig. 15.7. Brunnerioma: A highly echogenic, polypoid tumor near the papilla of Vater is seen.

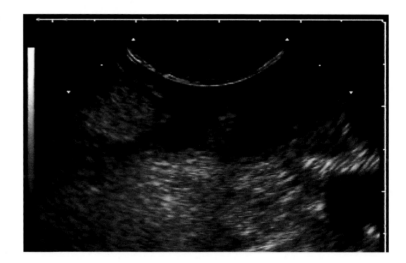

Fig. 15.8. Accessory spleen. The EUS transducer is located in the gastric fundus. An oval mass with smooth margins and a homogeneous echo pattern is found next to the pancreatic tail. It is clearly distinct from the pancreatic parenchyma. The differential diagnosis includes neuroendocrine tumors of the pancreas, tumors of the adrenal gland, and an accessory spleen. The isoechogenic pattern compared to the spleen and the location in front of the splenic vein support the diagnosis of an accessory spleen.

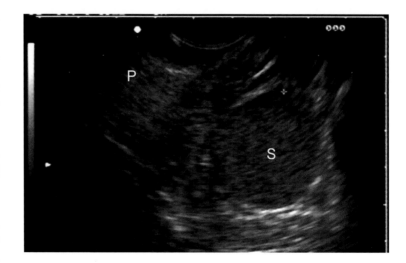

PART 4

Diagnostic Fine-Needle Biopsy

(For abbreviations see page 175)

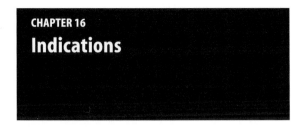

CHAPTER 16
Indications

P. Vilmann · G. K. Jacobsen

(For abbreviations see page 175)

Endoscopic ultrasound guided biopsy is increasingly being recognized as an integral part of an endoscopic ultrasound examination when a potentially malignant lesion is detected. Several publications have demonstrated that endoscopic ultrasound guided fine needle aspiration biopsy (EUS-FNA) is possible in most cases (Wiersema 1997; Vilmann 1998). Lesions in the gastrointestinal wall itself as well as lesions located adjacent to the wall may be punctured through the esophagus, stomach, duodenum or via the rectum. EUS-FNA is a relatively new technique which seems to have an important impact on therapeutic decision making. It is therefore necessary to critically evaluate the outcomes of EUS-FNA as well as to define its limitations and complications in order to define the exact indications of the technique.

When a decision is made to acquire equipment for EUS-FNA, one should be aware that a great deal of time has to be invested in this diagnostic method. The procedure is rather technically demanding and expertise is only acquired over time. Endosonography and EUS-FNA are traditionally performed by gastroenterologists. However, the close proximity of the GI tract to organs primarily of interest to other specialities makes them additional targets for EUS-FNA and one should expect requests for the examination from other specialities.

The indications for EUS guided biopsy are not fully known at present and will be determined only after randomized trials have compared it to conventional modalities. However, there is no doubt that the role of endosonography has expanded beyond the "staging of malignant GI-tumors" to include the diagnosis of previously undiagnosed primary lesions. In Table 16.1 and 16.2, diagnostic possibilities of EUS-FNA are listed which may predict its potential future role.

The following suggestions as to the indications for EUS-FNA are based on our personal experience with the procedure since 1991. Generally, EUS-FNA is reasonable in patients with lesions suggestive of malignancy in which standard approaches of obtaining a tissue diagnosis are unsuccessful or risky. It also seems reasonable to perform FNA in patients with lesions suggestive of malignancy that are detected only by EUS especially if an aspirate positive for malignancy will change patient management. Whether an aspirate positive for malignancy will change patient management varies among institutions throughout the world in our experience. Therefore, a close collaboration with the different specialities involved in each institution is essential, since the endosonographist in each case has to decide whether or not to perform FNA. The general indications established at Gentofte University Hospital are listed in Table 16.3.

Table 16.1. Primary diagnoses that may be obtained by EUS-FNA

Location	Type of lesion	Diagnosis
Mediastinum	Primary tumors	Esophageal cancer Submucosal tumors of the esophagus: leiomyoma and leiomyosarcoma or other stromal tumors, lymphomas Mesotheliomas Thymoma Lung cancer
	Lymph nodes	Metastases from undiagnosed primary tumors: breast cancer, gynecological cancer, GI cancer, lung cancer or other miscellaneous cancers Lymphomas Sarcoidosis Histoplasmosis Tuberculosis
Abdomen	Primary and secondary tumors	Gastric and duodenal tumors: carcinomas, submucosal stromal tumors and lymphomas Pancreatic tumors: carcinomas, neuroendocrine tumors Primary hepatobiliary tumors: hepatocellular carcinomas and biliary carcinomas Liver metastases Submucal tumors of the rectum Miscellaneous: primary and secondary tumors of the adrenal glands, the prostate and seminal vesicles
	Lymph nodes	Metastases from undiagnosed primary tumors - breast cancer, gynecological cancer, GI cancer, lung cancer, prostatic cancer and miscellaneous cancers Lymphomas Miscellaneous: sarcoidosis, histoplasmosis, tuberculosis

Table 16.2. Cancers in which EUS-FNA may have an important role in staging prior to therapy. FNA is mainly used to confirm N+ and M+ stage …

Location	Lymph nodes or metastases to organs	Diagnosis
Mediastinum	Staging	Lung cancer GI cancer: esophageal cancer, gastric cancer, pancreatic cancer Lymphomas Miscellaneous: gynecological cancer, urological cancer, breast cancer
Abdomen	Staging	Esophageal cancer Gastric and duodenal cancer Pancreatic cancer and malignant neuroendocrine tumors Hepatobiliary cancer Lymphomas Miscellaneous: urological cancer, gynecological cancer, breast cancer

Table 16.3. Indications for EUS-FNA established at Gentofte University Hospital

I.   Diagnosis of primary mediastinal tumors
II. Diagnosis of lung cancer or mesothelioma visualized by CT or MRI, located adjacent to the esophagus and not diagnosed by conventional biopsy methods
III. Diagnosis of lung cancer invasion of the mediastinum (Stage T-4)
IV. Lymph node staging in patients with malignant tumors if clinically relevant before therapeutic intervention (lung cancer, esophageal cancer, gastric cancer, pancreatic cancer, rectal cancer, gynecological cancer, urological cancer)
V.   Diagnosis of primary mucosal or submucosal tumors not diagnosed by conventional methods
VI. Diagnosis of local submucosal cancer recurrence (esophageal, gastric and rectal cancer)
VII. Diagnosis of lymph node enlargement visualized by other imaging techniques, such as CT, US or MR if undiagnosed by conventional methods
VIII. Diagnosis of suspected malignant pancreatic lesions not visible by conventional methods
IX. Diagnosis of neuroendocrine tumors of the pancreas not diagnosed by conventional methods
X.   Diagnosis of tumors in organs adjacent to the GI tract not diagnosed by conventional methods, i.e., adrenal glands, the liver, the prostate and the lower genito-urinary tract
XI. Diagnosis of fluid collections in patients with suspicion of carcinomatous ascites, malignant pleural effusion or malignant cysts

Diagnosis of Mediastinal Tumors Not Diagnosed by Conventional Biopsy Methods

Primary tumors located in the mediastinum adjacent to the esophagus are easy to diagnose with EUS-FNA in most cases. The lesion is most often visualized by either chest x-ray, CT or MR (Fig. 16.1). Our own experience includes a relatively large group of patients and this is without a doubt one of the major indications for EUS-FNA. These patients either have a primary mediastinal tumor, lung cancer (Fig. 16.2) or a mesothelioma (Figs. 16.3, 16.4) not diagnosed by conventional biopsy methods. Many of

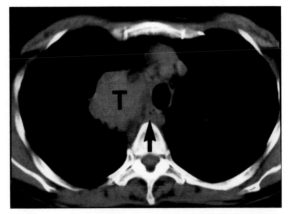

Fig. 16.1. Lung cancer demonstrated by computed tomography of the mediastinum. The tumor lies adjacent to the esophagus. *T*, Tumor; *arrow*, esophagus

Fig. 16.2. Transesophageal EUS guided biopsy of a hypoechoic tumor of the mediastinum. Note the reflections from the needle (*arrows*).

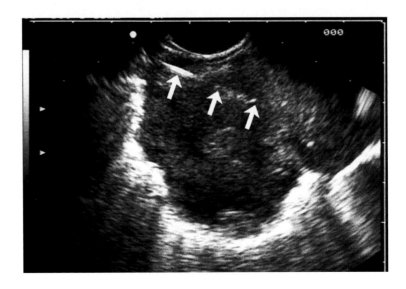

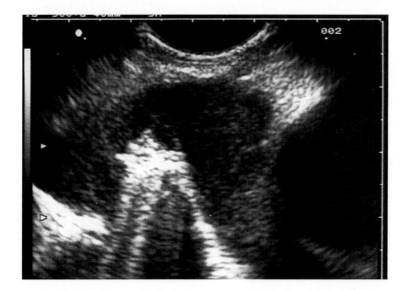

Fig. 16.3. Hypoechoic lesion of the mediastinal pleura compatible with a mesothelioma.

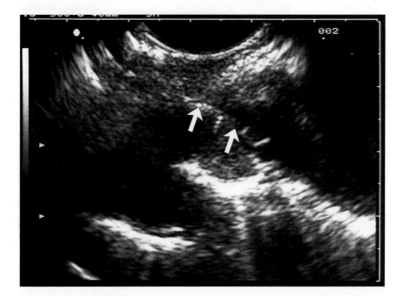

Fig. 16.4. Transesophageal EUS guided biopsy of an hypoechoic mesothelioma (arrows delineate the needle).

our patients are referred immediately prior to a planned explorative thoracotomy because other modalities such as mediastinoscopy and bronchoscopy with biopsy, or even trans-thoracic biopsy, were negative. If properly selected, these cases can be easily diagnosed. In many cases, a differentiation between non-small cell and small cell lung carcinoma, squamous cell carcinoma and adenocarcinoma is possible. Cost-benefit considerations are un-guestionably in favor of EUS-FNA, as many futile diagnostic explorations are avoided. A growing interest from pulmonary physicians who are becoming aware of this technique may be anticipated in the future.

Fig. 16.5. Lung cancer invasion of the mediastinum. Hypoechoic tumor is seen invading the aortopulmonary window. *AA*, Aortic arch; *LPA/(LPUA)*, left pulmonary artery; *TU*, tumor

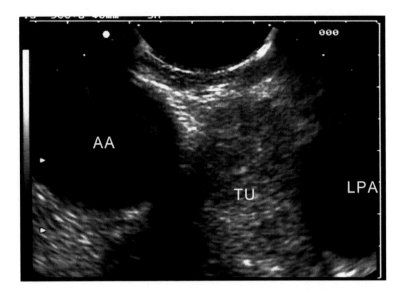

Fig. 16.6. Transesophageal EUS guided biopsy. Reflections from the needle are visualized as it penetrates the tumor (*arrows*).

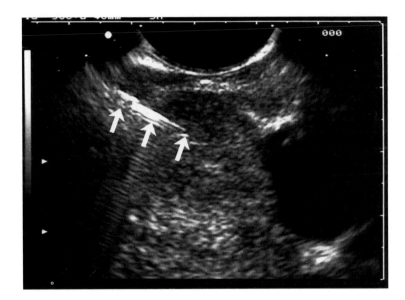

Diagnosis of Lung Cancer Invasion of the Mediastinum

Patients with previously diagnosed lung cancer who are considered candidates for surgery in whom CT or MR has demonstrated possible invasion of the mediastinum (Stage T4) are also often referred for EUS-FNA. In many of these cases, proof of unresectability as well as incurability can be obtained by cytology (Figs. 16.5, 16.6). Occasionally, a suspected invasion is rendered unlikely by a negative biopsy result.

Lymph Node Staging in Patients with Malignant Tumors

EUS-FNA of lymph nodes done for staging in patients with malignant tumors is indicated if a positive biopsy is considered clinically relevant before a final therapeutic intervention. This is one of the important indications for EUS-FNA, but the judgment on whether a positive biopsy is clinically relevant for the planning of therapy may differ from hospital to hospital. At our hospital, a biopsy demonstrating cancer in a contra-lateral lymph

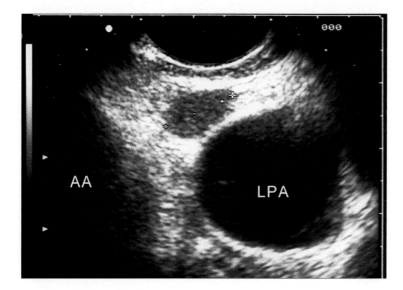

Fig. 16.7. A 1.2 cm lymph node located in the aortopulmonary window in a patient with lung cancer. *AA*, Aortic arch; *LPA/(LPUA)*, left pulmonary artery

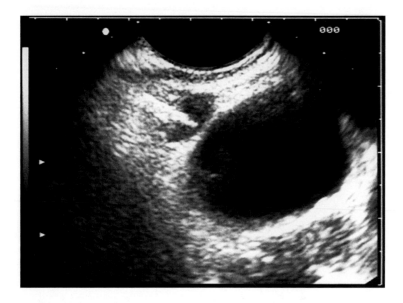

Fig. 16.8. Transesophageal biopsy of a 1.2 cm lymph node in the aortopulmonary window in a patient with lung cancer.

node or in a lymph node located in the subcarinal area in a lung cancer patient would exclude that patient from surgery (Figs. 16.7, 16.8). In these patients, a FNA of the lymph node in question is performed. In patients with esophageal cancer, only lymph node metastases regarded as distant metastases are biopsied. If a positive biopsy is obtained, the patient would be offered palliative therapy instead of resection. An example of this would be a patient with a squamous cell carcinoma of the esophagus and a lymph node metastasis at the celiac axis (Fig. 16.9). In most cases of gastric cancer,

a positive lymph node biopsy will not change patient management at our hospital, as many of these patients are offered resection. However, if a lymph node is visualized far from the primary lesion, as this may be regarded as a distant metastasis, EUS-FNA is performed. Occasionally, multiple lymph nodes in an elderly patient may lead the physician to opt for conservative measures. In patients with pancreatic cancer and lymph node metastases, an EUS-FNA is always indicated in our experience as no long term survivors are seen among these patients after surgical resection. In patients with rectal cancer and

Fig. 16.9. A 2 cm lymph node located in the arla of the celiac axis in a patient with esophageal cancer. EUS guided biopsy demonstrated a metastasis from a squamous cell carcinoma. *Arrow,* celiac axis

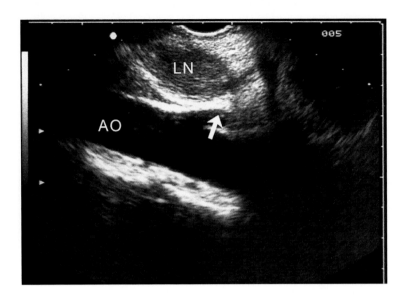

local lymph node metastases, a positive biopsy will occasionally change patient management to neo-adjuvant chemo-radiation therapy. Sometimes, a patient with gynecological cancer or urological cancer is referred to EUS-FNA after a CT scan has demonstrated lymph node enlargement adjacent to the upper GI tract. It is of great importance that a close collaboration between the referring physician and the endosonographer exists.

At present most patients from non-gastroenterological specialities are referred for a staging procedure only after other imaging techniques such as US, MR or CT have demonstrated enlarged lymph nodes suspicious for malignancy. An interesting question is whether EUS-FNA is of additional value in patients with cancers in whom conventional methods do not visualize lymph node enlargement. According to our experience, we routinely see such patients. Examination of such patients would, however, increase the number of patients referred considerably. At present, exams for this indication are not performed at our hospital. Hopefully, future studies will provide an answer to this question.

Diagnosis of Mucosal and Submucosal Tumors

Mucosal and submucosal tumors not diagnosed by conventional methods may also be considered for EUS-FNA. Occasionally, a patient is referred for EUS-FNA with a stenotic tumor of the esophagus in which conventional endoscopic biopsies have failed to diagnose the tumor. In most cases, the tumor can be visualized in full due to the longitudinal orientation of the transducer even if not traversable by the endoscope. EUS-FNA is not very difficult in these cases. In other cases, patients are referred for EUS-FNA with the suspicion of local anastomotic cancer recurrence after surgery done for esophageal, gastric or rectal cancer. Our policy is to begin with conventional endoscopic forceps biopsies. If these fail to diagnose a suspected recurrence, EUS-FNA is performed. Submucosal tumors may also be diagnosed by EUS-FNA, but the diagnostic success depends on the nature of the tumor (Fig. 16.10). Leiomyomas and leiomyosarcomas are difficult to diagnose. Even though spindle cells are collected, it may be difficult to differentiate whether the tumor is malignant or benign (Fig. 16.11). However, submucosal tumors may also be of a non-stromal type and in these cases, the diagnosis may be easy to obtain. Examples of such tumors are submucosal lymphomas.

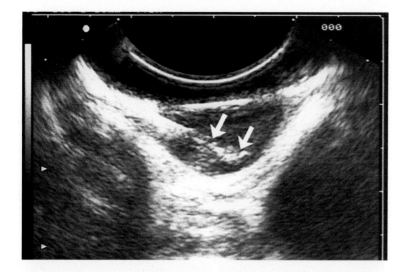

Fig. 16.10. EUS guided biopsy of a 2 cm submucosal tumor in the wall of the esophagus. *Arrows*, needle echo.

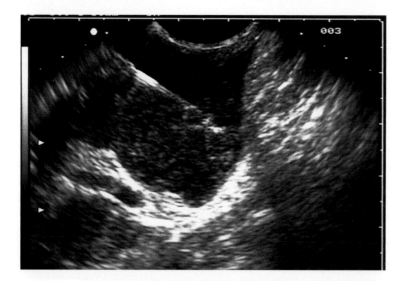

Fig. 16.11. EUS guided biopsy of a recurrent leiomyosarcoma of the stomach wall. The tumor is hypoechoic. Reflections from the needle can be seen in the tumor during the puncture.

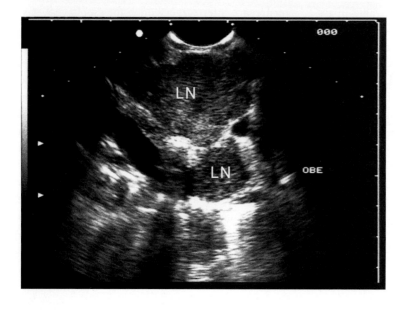

Fig. 16.12. Multiple lymph node metastases in the mediastinum in a patient with recurrent breast cancer. *LN*, Lymph nodes

Fig. 16.13. Transesophageal EUS guided biopsy of an enlarged lymph node in the mediastinum in the same patient as in Fig. 16.12. *Arrows*, reflections from the needle inside a lymph node.

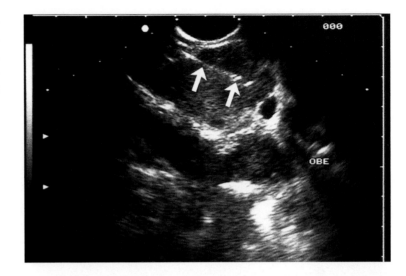

Fig. 16.14. A hypoechoic irregular lesion 4 cm in size located in the head of the pancreas that was not diagnosed by conventional methods. *TU*, Lesion

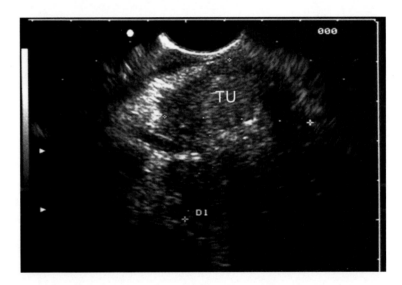

Differential Diagnosis of Lymph Node Enlargement Visualized by Other Imaging Techniques

In patients where other imaging techniques such as CT, US, or MR have diagnosed lymph node enlargement, EUS-FNA may be indicated if these lymph nodes are located adjacent to the GI-tract (Figs. 16.12, 16.13). Our policy is to try conventional biopsy methods first, if possible. If these attempts fail or if the lymph node is in a location where conventional biopsy cannot be done, EUS-FNA is performed. With this approach, metastases from undiagnosed cancers, lymphomas, histoplasmosis, tuberculosis and sarcoidosis have been diagnosed.

Diagnosis of Pancreatic Lesions Suspected of Malignancy

Patients with pancreatic tumors not visible on conventional methods are frequently referred for EUS-FNA. Some of these patients have small periampullary tumors or tumors of the papilla of Vater, and EUS-FNA is advantageous since these tumors are difficult to diagnose by other modalities. In our experience, even tumors of 2–4 cm in diameter may not be clearly visible by CT or US in all cases and these patients are also referred for EUS-FNA (Figs. 16.14, 16.15). Our policy is to perform EUS-FNA in patients where transcutaneous ultrasound has failed to diagnose a pancreatic lesion even if the

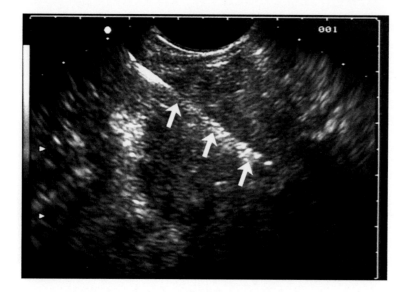

Fig. 16.15. Transduodenal biopsy of a 4-cm hypoechoic tumor in the head of the pancreas. *Arrows*, reflections from the needle during biopsy.

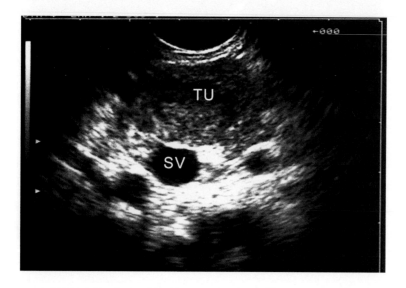

Fig. 16.16. Neuroendocrine tumor 2 cm in size at the tail of the pancreas that was not visualized by conventional imaging methods. *TU*, Tumor; *SV*, splenic vein

pancreas was clearly outlined by transcutaneous ultrasound scanning.

Diagnosis of Neuroendocrine Tumors of the Pancreas

Patients suspected of neuroendocrine tumors of the pancreas and not diagnosed by conventional methods are also considered for EUS-FNA at our department (Figs. 16.16, 16.17). These tumors may be insulinomas, gastrinomas, carcinoid tumors and others. Insulinomas and gastrinomas as small as 5 mm have been diagnosed by this technique. For planning of

therapy, the exact location of a neuroendocrine tumor is mandatory. If the suspected neuroendocrine tumor is not verified by EUS-FNA, an intraoperative US with intraoperative biopsy is considered before resection is started.

Diagnosis of Tumors in Organs Adjacent to the GI Tract and Not Diagnosed by Conventional Methods

EUS-FNA of tumors in other organs located adjacent to the GI tract may also be considered if not

Fig. 16.17. Transgastric EUS guided biopsy of a 2 cm neuroendocrine tumor in the tail of the pancreas. *Arrows*, reflections from needle.

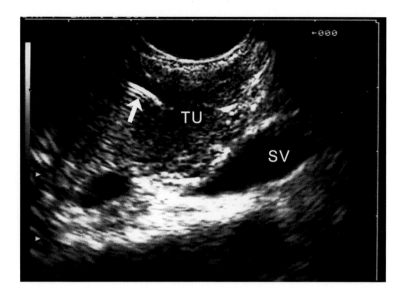

Fig. 16.18. Tumor of the left adrenal gland measuring 3 cm in size. *K*, Left kidney

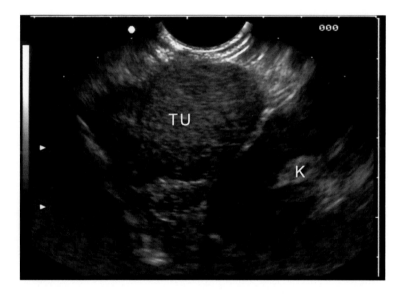

sucessfully diagnosed by conventional methods. At the present time it is difficult to exactly define the indications of EUS-FNA regarding these tumors. However, from time to time patients with lesions of the adrenal glands and the liver are diagnosed by this method (Figs. 16.18, 16.19). A lesion may have been visualized by CT or US, but it may be difficult to approach with transcutaneous biopsy. Alternatively, an unrecognized lesion may be seen during an EUS examination. It should be kept in mind that a lesion of the adrenals may be a pheocromocytoma. FNA is contraindicated in these cases. A pheocromocytoma should be evaluated for with urinalysis before EUS-

FNA. If a metastatic tumor of the adrenal is suspected, we perform biopsy without delay. Usually liver lesions are biopsied by the trancutaneous approach, but occasionally small unrecognized metastases in the left lobe of the liver are encountered during an EUS examination (Fig. 16.20). If so, EUS-FNA is done and, in most cases, confirmation of metastatic cancer can be made. Even hepatocellulary carcinoma may be diagnosed if the lesion is outlined by EUS. Theoretically, lower genitourinary tract lesions such as prostatic tumors may be reached by EUS-FNA, although most of these tumors are approached with rigid transrectal transducers at our institution.

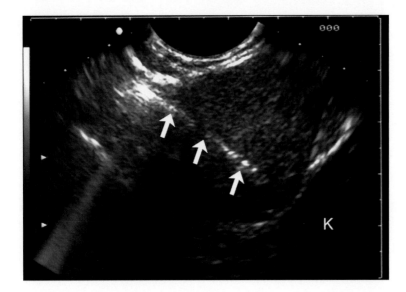

Fig. 16.19. A transgastric EUS guided biopsy of a 3 cm tumor of the left adrenal gland. *K*, Left kidney; *arrows*, reflections from needle.

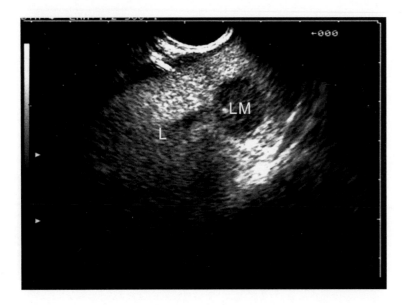

Fig. 16.20. EUS guided biopsy of a 1.3 cm metastasis in the left lobe of the liver. *L*, Liver; *LM*, liver metastasis.

Fig. 16.21. EUS guided aspiration of ascitic fluid in a patient with gastric cancer. *L*, Liver; *ST*, stomach wall; *arrow*, needle tip.

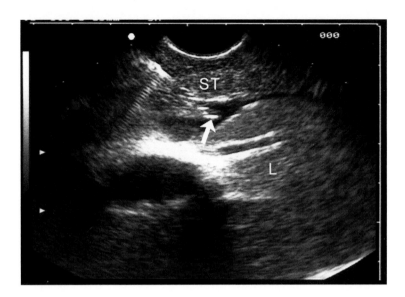

Fig. 16.22. EUS guided aspiration of fluid in a pancreatic cyst. The needle (*arrows*) is seen in the anechoic cyst (*CYS*).

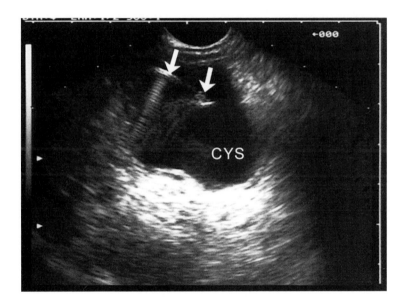

Diagnosis of Fluid Collections

If ascites or a pleural effusion is seen during an EUS examination in a patient with cancer, carcinomatosis should be suspected. Frequently, small fluid collections not recognized by other imaging modalities are seen. In this case, EUS guided fine needle aspiration is performed (Fig. 16.21). If malignant cells are seen in the fluid, carcinomatosis is verified and the patient is not a candidate for surgical resection.

Pancreatic cysts suspected of malignancy are punctured during EUS examination and the fluid is sent for measurement of the amylase concentration, cancer markers, and the presence of malignant cells (Fig. 16.22). When cysts are punctured, the patients should always be given antibiotics to reduce the risk of infection.

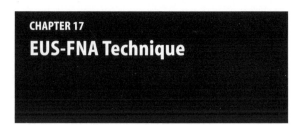

CHAPTER 17
EUS-FNA Technique

P. Vilmann · G.K. Jacobsen

Choice of Endoscope for EUS-FNA

At present, different endoscope models are available for performing EUS-FNA. The beginner is faced with several choices. Most endoscopists will, based on their own experience with conventional endoscopes, believe that a FNA endoscope with an elevator is preferable. The possibility of increasing the angle of the needle into a deeper position seems advantageous, but there are some draw-backs to this, in our experience. First, an elevator incorporated into the endoscope increases the length of the elongated stiff part of the distal end of the endoscope. This results in more difficulty in the maneuvering of the endoscope. Second, the additional force that the elevator exerts on the needle at their point of contact makes back and forth movement of the needle somewhat more difficult. We prefer instruments without elevators. Instead, we prefer echoendoscopes with a biopsy channel that is constructed with a predefined angle at the distal end of the endoscope.

Needles

In preliminary studies, needles employed in EUS-FNA were conventional needles such as used for sclerotherapy of esophageal varices or for trans-bronchial biopsy. However, these needles have been abandoned and are now considered inadequate for EUS-FNA, mainly due to their lack of stability and stiffness. At present, needles made entirely from steel containing a stylet are recommended so that the energy applied to the proximal end of the needle during puncture is sufficiently translated to the distal needle tip. This allows for penetration of hard lesions.

From 1991 to 1994, a special biopsy instrument with a handle device (GIP-Medizin Technik/Medi-Globe Corp., Type Hancke/Vilmann) was constructed by the authors in collaboration with their ultrasonic laboratory. It consists of a full length steel needle with a stylet, a metal spiral sheath, and a biopsy handle with a piston (Fig. 17.1). The special

Fig. 17.1. Biopsy handle instrument (GIP Medizin Technique/ MediGlobe). *A*, Needle with stylet screw fixated to the piston; *B*, lock button; *C*, metal spiral sheath screw fixed to the biopsy handle

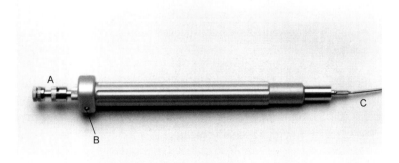

biopsy instrument with a handle device was primarily developed for a curved array echoendoscope (Pentax FG-32 UA) and its successors, such as the Pentax FG-34 UX. However it can also be used in conjunction with other puncture echoendoscopes. This biopsy instrument is considered the best and most safe system for EUS-FNA available at the moment, and most studies today are performed with this instrument.

The steel needle has a length of 170 cm and has an outer diameter of 0.8 mm (G 22). The needle tip is sharp and tapered to a point, and its distal end has been sand blasted to improve ultrasonic visualization. The needle can be luerlocked to the handle piston. A stylet, which can be luerlocked to the proximal end of the needle, ends approximately 5 mm beyond the needle tip when in place. Its distal end is rounded. The blunt-tipped stylet was constructed for safety reasons to avoid puncture of the endoscope during introduction of the needle into the working channel of the endoscope.

A needle with a larger diameter of 19 G (1 mm) is also available but this needle can only be used in endoscopes with larger biopsy channels than the Pentax FG-32 UA or FG-34 UX (i. e. more than 2 mm in diameter). At present, three such curved linear array echoendoscopes are commercially available: the Pentax FG-36 UX, the Pentax FG-38 UX, and the Olympus GF UC30P.

The metal spiral sheath housing the AG needle is 138 centimeters long, 1.8 millimeters in outer diameter, and can be screw-fixated to the distal outlet of the biopsy handle. When fully inserted into the endoscope, the spiral sheath ends 0.5 to 1.0 centimeters beyond the distal end of the biopsy channel (Fig. 17.2). Because of different lengths of biopsy channels of different types of endoscopes, a need for different lengths of needles and sheath's has arisen. As a result, these have become commercially available.

The biopsy handle consists of an aluminum cylinder and a stainless steel piston. The piston can be moved back and forth within the handle cylinder. Inside the handle cylinder, the piston has a telescopic construction supporting the needle. A special locking system with a button on the proximal end of the handle cylinder secures the piston and the needle in a withdrawn position. The locked position of the piston can be released by pressing the button. The special button locking system on the handle cylinder

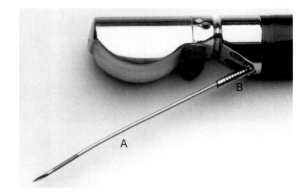

Fig. 17.2. Distal end of a curved array echo endoscope (Pentax FG 32 UA) with the GIP needle. *A*, Needle; *B*, metal spiral sheath

is primarily for the protection of the channel of the endoscope against damage. The piston, when locked in a withdrawn position, prevents the needle from being advanced unintentionally during the introduction of the sheath and the needle into the biopsy channel. It also is protective during the necessary transducer manoeuvring immediately before the FNA puncture.

For full assembly, the spiral sheath is first screwed onto the handle cylinder, and the needle with the stylet then inserted via the handle piston and luerlocked to its proximal end. Finally the handle cylinder can be luerlocked to the inlet of the biopsy channel of the endoscope (Fig. 17.3).

The needle can be advanced up to 10 cm beyond the metal sheath by pushing the handle piston into the handle. By anchoring the handle to the inlet of the biopsy channel of the endoscope, the power applied to the handle piston is directly transmitted to the needle tip. Additionally, the outer metal sheath is secured in a fixed position to avoid advancement of the sheath more distally than desired. Consequently, penetration of the gut wall with the sheath is not possible. The sheath secured in a fixed position also protects the biopsy channel during back and forth movements of the steel needle, so that the endoscope damage previously described can be avoided.

At present, three other aspiration needle systems are commercially available which are constructed in similar fashion. Two of these are disposable needle sets (GIP-Medizin Technik/Medi-Globe Corp and Wilson-Cook) (Figs. 17.4, 17.5). The GIP-needle, in addition, has the possibility of adjusting the length

Fig. 17.3. The biopsy handle instrument (GIP Medizin Technique/MediGlobe) luer-locked to the inlet of the biopsy channel of the endoscope (Pentax FG 32 UA). The piston (*A*) is retracted so that the biopsy handle is ready for puncture.

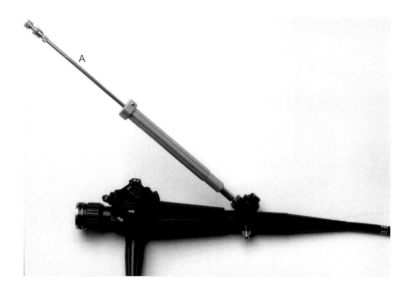

Fig. 17.4. Disposable biopsy handle instrument for EUS guided biopsy (GIP Medizin Technique/MediGlobe). The length of the metal spiral sheath can be adjusted by a screw mechanism incorporated in the handle. *A*, Biopsy handle; *B*, metal spiral sheath and needle; *C*, screw for adjustment of the metal spiral sheath length.

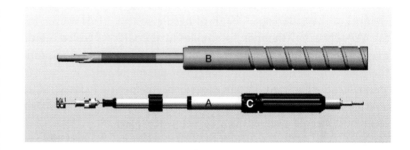

Fig. 17.5. Disposable biopsy handle instrument for EUS guided biopsy (Wilson-Cook). *A*, Biopsy handle; *B*, syringe for aspiration.

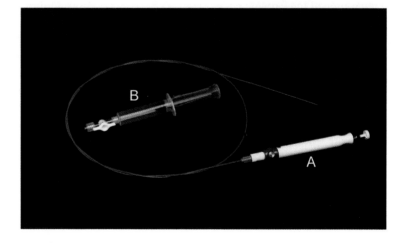

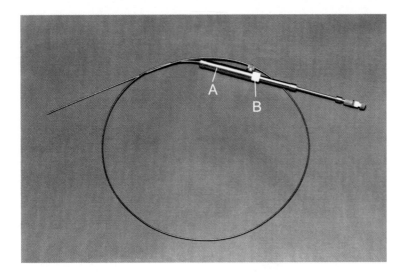

Fig. 17.6. Biopsy handle instrument for EUS guided biopsy (Olympus). *A*, Biopsy handle; *B*, screw for adjustment of the length of the metal spiral sheath.

of its metal spiral sheath to the length of the biopsy channel of the endoscope. The third needle system for EUS-FNA, by Olympus, is similar to the GIP needle system (Type Hancke/Vilmann). It also has the possibility of adjusting the length of the metal spiral sheath (Fig. 17.6). In our experience, disposable needle systems are not as stable as the multiple use biopsy needle systems. As a consequence, hard tumors may be difficult to penetrate with the disposable needles.

Preparation of the Patient

Under normal conditions, sedatives and topical pharyngeal anesthetics are used in EUS-FNA as in conventional endoscopy . In most cases, the biopsy can be done without any additional discomfort to the patient and analgesics are seldom necessary. However, patients with pancreatic lesions (especially those with advanced lesions) may benefit from a strong analgesic given intravenously before the biopsy. In rare cases where complete relaxation is desired, either because of difficult localization or targeting of the lesion, general anesthesia may be recommend.

Laboratory tests are not routinely required, and the procedure is performed on an outpatient basis. In selected patients with impaired liver function or on anticoagulation therapy, measuring the prothrombin time and the platelet count prior to the procedure is advisable.

Prophylactic antibiotics are not routinely used. However, in patients in whom puncture of a cystic lesion is indicated or a lesion is biopsied through the rectum, antibiotics are recommended.

EUS-FNA: General Procedure

First, the target is clearly outlined by EUS. If available, color Doppler examination of the target lesion as well as the path that the needle is expected to traverse should be performed. In our experience, this additional data may prevent unintended puncture of interposed vessels and highly vascularized tumors occasionally encountered.

The transducer must constantly be held in firm contact with the GI wall during puncture. This is recommended during all EUS-FNA procedures, regardless of the exact location of the lesion. The needle is then inserted into the working channel of the endoscope. Immediately before the biopsy is performed, the transducer position is chosen so that it brings the puncture target and the needle route into focus. This may be accomplished by deflection of the tip of the endoscope, whereby the lesion is lifted up in the ultrasonic image (Figs. 17.7, 17.8). This procedure is particularly important for biopsy of deep extraluminal lesions. The needle is then advanced so that the reflections of the needle tip are seen on EUS. The needle tip is pushed against the GI wall and the stylet is withdrawn a few millimeters in order to expose the sharp needle tip. The needle,

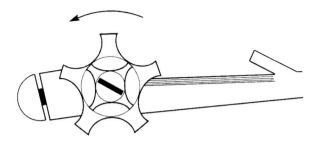

Fig. 17.7. Illustration of the procedure of deflection of the distal end of the endoscope and transducer. This brings the FNA target into the path of the needle.

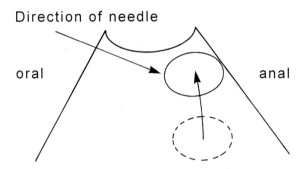

Fig. 17.8. Illustration of an imaginary lesion in an ultrasonic sectional image. By deflecting the distal end of the endoscope, the lesion outlined by endosonography is lifted up in the ultrasonic image.

containing the partially withdrawn stylet, is then advanced into the lesion under constant ultrasound guidance. The stylet is then removed completely. Some authors recommend that the stylet is repositioned before it is withdrawn, in order to remove the primary tissue plug consisting of superficial layers of the GI-wall from the needle. Suction is then applied through the needle by means of a 10 or 20 ml syringe; some authors perform FNA without suction which can be helpful in larger and soft lesion where aspiration may lead to specimens containing too much blood. The needle is further advanced into the lesion and moved back and forth under ultrasound monitoring. Between 5 and 10 back and forth movements within the lesion are sufficient. The suction is then equilibrated while the tip of the needle is still in the lesion. The needle is now withdrawn, and the needle and the catheter are removed. The aspirated material is subsequently expelled and smeared onto glass slides.

Complete needle visualization should be the goal in every biopsy in order to prevent unintended puncture of vessels. In our experience, adequate needle visualization also increases the sensitivity of the biopsy compared to punctures without full needle visualization.

EUS-FNA: Procedure with the Special Biopsy Instrument with a Handle Device

1. The biopsy instrument is assembled, and the handle piston is locked in a withdrawn position.
2. The spiral sheath with the needle and stylet is introduced through the biopsy channel of the endoscope, and the handle cylinder is screwed onto the inlet of the biopsy channel.
3. After the puncture target is adequately visualized by EUS, the locking system of the handle is released by pressing the button, and the needle with the stylet is advanced beyond the end of the metal sheath and pressed firmly against the target by pushing the handle piston. Reflections from the needle can then be seen on EUS.
4. The stylet is unlocked and withdrawn 5 millimeters to expose the sharp needle and to avoid plugging up the needle with mucosal cells.
5. The needle with the stylet is advanced into the lesion under EUS guidance by pushing the handle piston.
6. The stylet is removed completely.
7. Suction is applied through the needle by means of a 10 or 20 ml syringe.
8. The needle is further advanced into the lesion and moved back and forth several times under continued EUS guidance.
9. The suction is released while the tip of the needle is still within the lesion.
10. The needle is withdrawn completely to a locked position by means of the handle piston.
11. The instrument is removed from the endoscope and the aspirated material is expelled and further processed as described.

In difficult cases, the endoscopist has to actively maintain the contact of the transducer to the GI wall during the needle puncture. Therefore, in these cases, an assistant should preferably introduce the needle and perform the aspiration. However, in most cases, the endoscopist can perform the biopsy with one hand while maneuvering the endoscope with the other hand. When inside the lesion, and after the stylet is removed, the aspiration is begun by an assistant or by an aspiration syringe (see Fig. 17.5).

Introduction of the needle into a lesion is most easily performed with the endoscope in a straight position, as is the case in the esophagus. However, puncture is also possible with the endoscope in a curved position such as when positioned in the second part of the duodenum. In cases where the tip of the endoscope is flexed maximally or where the endoscope has a loop, the instrument should be deflected until needle passage is possible.

It is important not to withdraw the stylet more than a few millimeters before puncture in order to avoid water or mucus being aspirated into the needle and to avoid tissue plugs, consisting of superficial layers of the GI-wall, obstructing the needle. The importance of a steady position of the transducer in relation to the lesion to be punctured should be stressed. When the needle is introduced through the GI wall, it seems relatively easy to hit the target. However, it may be difficult to keep the transducer in constant contact with the GI wall because the wall and surrounding structures have a tendency to move and the transducer has a tendency to change its position when needle puncture is performed. In cases of inadequate needle monitoring, the needle is at first withdrawn to a point just beneath the transducer, corresponding to a position only a few centimeters beyond the biopsy channel. If the needle is not fully visible by then, the needle is withdrawn completely and a new step-by-step FNA procedure as described above is again initiated.

There is a tendency to lose ultrasound contact with the needle tip, particularly when hard lesions are penetrated. This, however, is not a major problem, since adjustment of the transducer position usually reestablishes ultrasound imaging of the needle rather easily.

Before removal of the needle it is mandatory to stop the suction completely. If this is not done, water or mucus will inevitably be sucked into the needle when removed. The aspirated material may consequently be destroyed.

Under normal circumstances, the entire biopsy procedure lasts between 5 and 15 minutes. The amount of time needed for the biopsy is dependent on the location of the target to be punctured. Biopsies from the esophagus are usually fast, taking about 5 minutes. Biopsies of firm lesions in the head of the pancreas can take up to 15 minutes.

EUS-FNA in the Esophagus

In the esophagus, the transducer is first placed directly onto the mucosa or onto the surface of the lesion to be biopsied. If the ultrasound coupling is insufficient, the balloon can be filled with a few ml of water just before needle introduction or immediately after the needle has gained contact with the mucosa. However, this is rarely necessary.

The position of the sheath and needle tip may be visualized through the optic lens before the needle advanced and further visualized by ultrasound. However, this is rarely necessary with the special biopsy instrument with a handle device because the metal sheath is always positioned just beyond the distal outlet of the biopsy channel when the biopsy handle is anchored to the inlet of the biopsy channel of the endoscope.

Generally EUS-FNA of lesions punctured via the esophagus is relatively easy since most of these lesions are soft and the endoscope is held in a straight position during the procedure. Biopsy through vessels should be avoided, but is seldom a problem.

Lesions located in the upper third of the esophagus such as lymph nodes along the vessels of the neck, primary esophageal lesions, or lesions located high in the superior mediastinum can be biopsied. However the proximal position of the transducer in the esophagus is very unpleasant and frequently results in an agitated and uncooperative patient. In these cases, general anesthesia is therefore preferable. Biopsies of lesions within the wall of the middle or distal third of the esophagus can usually be done even in cases of total stenosis. Lesions in the mediastinum such as lymph nodes, primary mediastinal tumors, and lung cancers located adjacent to the esophagus can also be biopsied. Most of the lymph nodes in the mediastinum are anatomically in close contact to the intra-thoracic part of the esophagus. The movement of the heart is rarely a problem, since the distance from the transducer to the lymph nodes of interest is short. This allows for biopsy of even very small lesions with a diameter of less than 1 cm.

EUS-FNA in the Stomach

In patients with pathological conditions of the stomach, acoustic coupling is either achieved by direct mucosa/transducer contact or by instillation of water into the stomach. Direct contact with the lesion is generally preferred even in cases where water instillation is used. This is because if the transducer is not placed directly against the lesion in the stomach wall, the transducer tends to be pushed away from the lesion when the needle is advanced for puncture. Lesions within the gastric wall are among the most difficult lesions to biopsy. Instead of maintaining its original position, the stomach wall tends to move back and forth with the needle movement, thus preventing the needle from only moving within the lesion as desired. In addition, many of these lesions are relatively firm and difficult to puncture.

The body and tail of the pancreas are punctured through the stomach. It is possible to biopsy lesions in the head of the pancreas from the antrum of the stomach or from the duodenal bulb. This is often done in cases where distal stenosis or obstruction is caused by the underlying lesion.

Also lymph nodes surrounding the stomach and lymph nodes located at the celiac axis, the splenic vessels, the splenic hilum, the left gastric artery, the hepatic artery, the hepato-duodenal ligament and the portal hilum can undergo FNA via the stomach. Even a biopsy of most parts of the left lobe of the liver can easily be accomplished through the gastric wall. Vessels interposed between the transducer and the target lesion may prevent biopsy. However, repositioning the transducer can often solve this problem. Patients with Klatskin tumors are typical examples of this situation, as the portal vein is often located between the transducer and the lesion. A shift of the transducer position to the first part of the duodenum may sometimes allow a FNA to be performed in this challenging situation.

In patients with a lesion in the fundus of the stomach, the lesion is either approached via the distal esophagus or the cardia. It may also be directly punctured from below with the endoscope in retroflexion. However, in the latter case, the endoscope has to be in a straight position when introducing the special biopsy instrument with a handle device. The endoscope is then retroflexed and the aspiration biopsy performed using direct transducer contact with the lesion as described previously.

EUS-FNA in the Duodenum

The head of the pancreas with the papilla of Vater is punctured from the second part of the duodenum with direct contact of the transducer with the duodenal wall. Due to a relatively curved position of the endoscope from the stomach to the second part of the duodenum, some resistance during needle movement is felt. Additionally, many solid lesions of the pancreas are relatively hard and forceful needle penetration may be necessary. As a result of this, the lesion and the pancreas tend to move back and forth with the needle movements. The transducer is sometimes even pushed away from the duodenal wall and adequate needle monitoring may be lost. If this happens, acoustic coupling may be regained by filling the balloon with water. It can also be of great help to have an assistant keeping the endoscope in position or even pushing it forward during the biopsy. Occasionally, it may be very difficult to maintain a steady transducer position in the second part of the duodenum, particularly in patients with large and hard lesions. Inflation of the balloon with water after advancing the needle into the lesion may help in these cases, since this may improve ultrasound coupling with the duodenal wall.

Lymph nodes inferior to the pancreatic head at the uncinate process can also be biopsied from the second or third part of the duodenum. Biopsies of lymph nodes cranially to the head of the pancreas and lesions in the liver hilum are done through the first part of the duodenum, the duodenal bulb, or even through the gastric antrum.

EUS-FNA in the Rectum

Lesions within the rectal wall as well as lesions outside of the rectal wall can undergo FNA. In most cases, the endoscope can be held in a straight position and biopsy is therefore relatively simple. This is especially true with regard to lymph nodes and extraluminal cancer recurrences.

CHAPTER 18

Cytopathology Interpretation

G.K. Jacobsen · P. Vilmann

Slide Preparation

The process begins with the aspirate being expelled onto glass slides. Even at this moment, a preliminary macroscopic evaluation of the material is possible. Material aspirated from a malignant lesion, usually a carcinoma, is often gray or yellow and finely granular. It can be necrotic and/or mucoid. Cystic lesions yield a thin liquid material. Thin bloody aspirates often do not contain diagnostic material. Aspirates from mesenchymal tumors may contain small cohesive clumps of tissue.

The aspirate should be spread on the glass slides in a uniformly thin layer or film in order to allow for examination by light microscopy. In our experience, the following technique using two glass slides results in optimal smears: After the aspirate has been expelled onto the glass slide another glass slide is placed upside down on top of the first slide. Without applying pressure, the glass slides are slowly moved in opposite directions. As a result the material is spread in a thin layer on both slides, resulting in two almost identical smears. If the material is very thick with clumps of material, some pressure with the second glass slide should be applied during the process.

The material can also be spread on the slide with the conventional method that hematologists often use, i.e. spreading the aspirate with a small coverglass with rounded edges.

After the material has been spread, it has to be further processed for microscopic evaluation. Two major methods are available. The smeared aspirate can either be fixed immediately or it can be air-dried. The decision of which method to use depends on the choice of staining method, the laboratory protocol, and the experience of the cytopathologist. For immediate fixation, commercially available solutions such as sprayfix, alcohol, and acetone can be applied, depending on the staining method. Air-drying, on the other hand, is easy to handle, very practical, and can be left without further fixation for months without degradation of the cells. All fixed or air-dried smears can be sent for further processing elsewhere if necessary.

If the aspiration yields a large amount of material, some of it may be expelled into formaldehyde, collected in a cell pellet, embedded in paraffin, and finally cut and stained for histological examination. Some authors prefer this method, as 80% of biopsies are core biopsies containing sufficient tissue fragments for histological evaluation. If indicated, the material can also be collected in special fixatives for electron-microscopic (EM) examination. However, in many cases where EM was previously used, it has now been replaced by immunohistochemical (IM) methods. Immunohistochemistry is usually done in tissue sections, but this method can also be applied to smears from aspirates.

Staining of the smears may be performed in various ways. Quick staining with Hemacolor (Mer.11661) can be done at the bedside. This offers the possibility to evaluate the quality of the material at once and make another aspirate, if necessary.

Immediately fixed smears are usually stained with hematoxylin and eosin (HE) or according to the Papanicoulau (PAP) protocol. Air-dried smears are generally stained according to the May-Grünwald-Giemsa protocol (MGM). The choice of staining technique is a matter of tradition, routine, and experience of the cytopathologist. MGM is widely used for FNA and yields excellent staining results with a distinct cell morphology, in our experience. MGM staining takes 15–20 minutes, and a diagnosis may be made within half an hour.

Special cytochemical staining for various substances such as melanin, iron and neurosecretory products can also be done. If the previously described two glass spreading method is used, one slide may be stained routinely, while the other is held back for special stains should they be necessary.

Microscopical Evaluation

The interpretation of EUS-FNA does not vary substantially from that of FNA obtained through other techniques (Figs. 19.1–19.6). There are, however, pitfalls which should be taken into consideration. First of all, contamination of the aspirate with cells from the esophagus is very common. This means that squamous cells from the surface epithelium of the esophagus are present in the aspirate in various numbers. Depending on the lesion and the origin of the EUS-FNA, such squamous cells may provoke a false diagnosis of a metastatic lesion. This is especially true if they are reactively altered and detected among cells from a lymph node.

Another problem is the interpretation of an EUS-FNA comprised of malignant and lymphatic cells. The cytopathologist can never tell with certainty whether the detected cells represent a primary lesion with additional cells from a lymphocytic infiltrate or lymph node or if they represent a secondary metastatic lesion within a lymph node. The interpretation of a FNA must be done in close cooperation with the clinician who performed the endoscopy and who knows the exact location of the needle when the aspirate was taken.

In aspirates from mesenchymal tumors, such as leiomyomas, the cellularity may be rather scant and the material may only be present in clumps and clusters. The morphology of the cells on the periphery of these clumps, however, is usually characteristic.

In conclusion, from the point of view of the cytopathologist, EUS-FNA is not much different from FNA in general. As in all cytopathological evaluations and interpretations, experience within the field is mandatory. In addition, close cooperation with the clinician performing the examination is essential.

Fig. 18.1. A cluster of **adenocarcinoma cells** is seen on a slightly blood-stained background. The aspirate is from the stomach wall. (MGM stain)

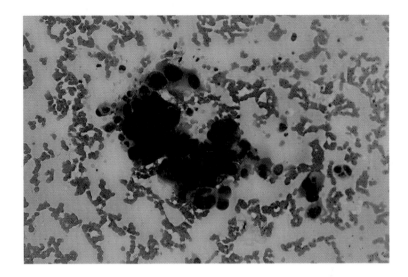

Fig. 18.2. A few **pleomorphic carcinoma cells** are seen among lymphocytic cells. In addition, a squamous cell from the surface epithelium of esophagus is present. The aspirate is from a lymph node with a metastasis from a poorly differentiated squamous cell carcinoma of the lung. (MGM stain)

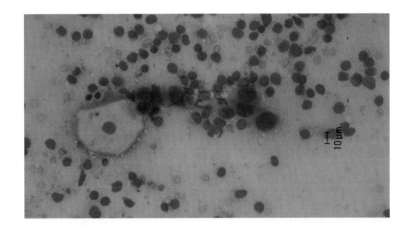

Fig. 18.3. Clusters of **mesenchymal cells** are seen on a clean background. The cells have typical elongated nuclei that are rather uniform. The aspirate is from a leiomyoma in the stomach wall. (MGM stain)

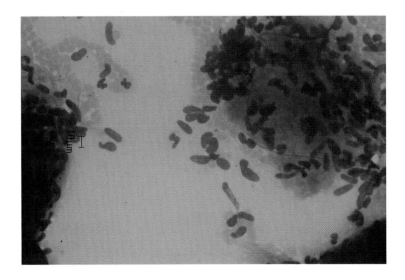

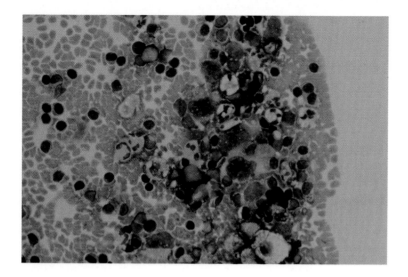

Fig. 18.4. A mixture of pleomorphic cells, lymphocytes, and blood is shown. The pleomorphic cells are obviously malignant, but the origin of the cells is difficult to determine. The material is from a mediastinal lymph node. (MGM stain)

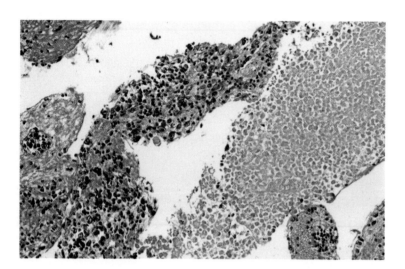

Fig. 18.5. A section from a cell **pellet obtained from the previous aspirate is seen.** Tightly packed, more or less preserved tumor cells are present to the left with necrotic cells to the right. (HE stain)

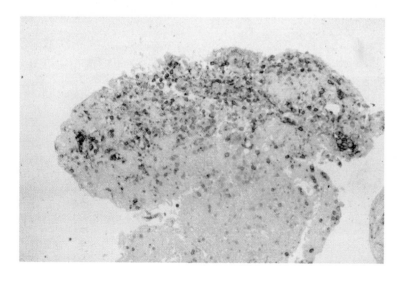

Fig. 18.6. Positive immunoperoxidase staining for lymphocytic common antigen (*LCA*) in the tumor cells in the same cell pellet is shown, indicating that the aspirate is from a malignant lymphoma. Further staining also demonstrated B-cell markers.

CHAPTER 19
EUS-FNA Study Results

P. Vilmann · G.K. Jacobsen

A rapidly expanding number of studies on EUS-FNA are being published. Most of these studies, however, were performed in specialized centers. Beginners have to overcome several challenges before acceptable diagnostic results can be expected. First, the interpretation of the difficult anatomy as seen with a curved linear array transducer has to be learned before EUS-FNA of different lesions can begin. Second, the biopsy technique has to be adequately mastered before sufficient material can be obtained from a lesion. Third, an experienced cytopathologist should be available for interpretation of the aspirates.

The overall sensitivity of EUS-FNA for malignant disease has been reported to be in the range of 80–85%, with a positive predictive value (PPV) of 100% and an accuracy between 80–90%. However, there are huge variations in success rates since the diagnostic values are highly dependent on both the site of the biopsy as well as the nature of the lesion that is being biopsied. Mediastinal tumors and lymph nodes yield the best results, with a sensitivity of more than 90%. This is followed by EUS-FNA of pancreatic lesions with a sensitivity between 80–85%. The diagnostic values also vary considerably with regard to the size of the lesion, but even FNA of lymph nodes less than 1 cm in diameter has a sensitivity of around 75% (Vilmann 1996, Wiersema 1997).

EUS guided Biopsy of Lesions Within the Gastrointestinal Wall

EUS guided biopsies of lesions within the gastrointestinal wall have the lowest diagnostic values and the highest rate of inconclusive biopsies. In our collaborative multicenter study with 457 patients and 554 lesions biopsied, 115 lesions were located within the GI wall. Twelve of these lesions were sub-mucosal tumors, five were localized in the esophagus and seven were in the stomach. The accuracy of EUS guided FNA cytology of submucosal tumors was 50%, with one half of the biopsy specimens being inadequate. In cases of smooth muscle tumors, although cytology demonstrated spindle cells in 4 of 7 cases, not a single case of a leiomyosarcoma was detected. EUS-FNA was performed on 103 non-stromal tumors localized in the gastrointestinal wall (esophagus 32, stomach 52, duodenum 10, rectum 9) with a sensitivity, specificity, PPV, NPV and accuracy of 61%, 79%, 100%, 76% and 67% respectively. The sensitivity of diagnosing gastric non-Hodgkins lymphoma (89%, 8/9) was better than diagnosing gastric adenocarcinoma (40%, 10/25). The accuracy of EUS-FNA for mucosal lesions in the esophagus was 69%. The accuracy of EUS-FNA for gastric, duodenal, and rectal muscusal lesions was 62%, 60%, and 100% respectively.

EUS guided Biopsy of Extraintestinal Lesions

The results of EUS guided FNA biopsy of extraintestinal mass lesions were described in the publication of the above mentioned multicenter study and included 139 patients with 145 lesions, of which 40 were found to be benign and 105 malignant. The site of the lesions included the liver (n=12), the pancreas (n=124), the abdomen (n=7), and the pelvic region (n=2). Within the subgroup of patients with hepatic, abdominal, or pelvic masses, 6 benign and 13 malignant lesions underwent EUS-FNA with a sensitivity, specificity and accuracy of 100%. EUS-FNA for pancreatic masses demonstrated a sensitivity of 86%, a specificity of 94%, a PPV of 100%, a NPV of 86%, and an accuracy of 88%.

Our own results of EUS-FNA in 85 patients with masses located in the mediastinum showed a sensitivity of 90% (unpublished data). In most of these patients, other diagnostic modalities had been inconclusive.

EUS Guided Biopsy of Lymph Nodes

One of the major advances of EUS-FNA appears to be an improvement in diagnosing malignant lymph nodes. Vilmann et al described their experience with lymph node biopsies in 44 patients with 47 lymph nodes (1996). The diameter of the lymph nodes ranged between 0.4 and 5 cm, with a mean of 1.5 cm. The mean number of passes per node was 1.5, with the range being from 1 to 4. The sensitivity of EUS-FNA in this study was 93%, and the specificity 100%. However, a relatively high rate of inconclusive biopsies was found (16%).

In the previously described multicenter study, EUS-FNA was performed on 192 lymph nodes in 171 patients. Forty-six lymph nodes were found to be benign on follow-up and 146 proved to be malignant. EUS guided FNA of lymph nodes demonstrated the best results compared to EUS guided FNA in extra-intestinal masses and gastrointestinal wall lesions with a sensitivity, specificity, PPV, NPV and accuracy of 92%, 93%, 100%, 86% and 92% respectively.

Reviewing the literature, sarcoidosis and mediastinal histoplasmosis have also been diagnosed by EUS guided biopsy.

CHAPTER 20

Limitations and Complications

P. Vilmann · G.K. Jacobsen

(For abbreviations see page 175)

As EUS-FNA is an interventional procedure and similar to other interventional procedures, there is a potential risk of complications from either the needle puncture itself or endoscopic manipulation. However, if risky procedures are avoided and basic principles are adhered to, EUS-FNA can be regarded as a safe procedure. In our multicenter study (Wiersema 1997*), complications were reported in up to 2% of the cases. Most of these were of a minor nature. Minor bleeding is always seen at the puncture site, but this is limited to a few ml in most cases. Major bleeding requiring surgery has been described in only a few cases. Perforation, mainly due to trying to advance the endoscope through a stenotic tumor may be seen. However, this cannot be regarded as a direct consequence of the biopsy procedure itself. Naturally, one should avoid maneuvering the endoscope with the biopsy needle already introduced, since the exposed part of the metal sheath may injure the gastrointestinal wall. Infections of cystic lesions are a potential problem and have been described in up to 14% of patients with pancreatic pseudocyst punctures. However, recent studies in which patients with pancreatic pseudocysts received antibiotics before FNA showed a significantly lower infection rate. Some cases of pancreatitis have been described after pancreatic biopsies. In most of these cases, however, only an elevation of s-amylase without clinically symptomatic pancreatitis was observed. Air embolism without any symptomatic consequence has been described in a single case. This is probably of no concern, so long as one avoids the injection of air during aspiration with the syringe. Tumor cell seeding after EUS-FNA, although not yet published, is a potential problem which has created some concern. However, as judged from results obtained from large studies with transcutaneous ultrasound guided FNA, tumor cell seeding seems to be a very limited problem. As a preventive method, biopsy through tumor infiltrated layers of the GI-wall should be avoided. A theoretical advantage of EUS-FNA compared to transcutaneous biopsy is the generally shorter needle tract. This tract is later resected in most cases, minimizing the risk of spreading malignant cells from the main lesion. An example is the preoperative biopsy of a malignant pancreatic head lesion undergoing a subsequent Whipple's resection.

With the development of EUS-FNA a new field has been created in endosonography. However, there are some limitations. Moving structures, such as lymph nodes moving with the heart beat or the aortic pulse, may be difficult to target and a puncture between two contractions may be necessary. A restless, uncooperative patient can make the biopsy hazardous. Also, minute tumors may be difficult to target and in combination with the above-mentioned difficulties, a successful biopsy is unlikely. In our experience, however, even neuroendocrine tumors as small as 5 mm have been diagnosed with EUS-FNA. However, we prefer to perform the biopsy with the patient under general anesthesia in these cases. The correct diagnosis of mesenchymal tumors such as leiomyomas and leiomyosarcomas is a problem that seems difficult to solve with EUS-FNA. Even though spindle cells can sometimes be collected, clear differentiation between benign and malignant tumors is difficult. This is mainly due to the fact that a definite malignant diagnosis can only be made on the basis of the histopathological examination of larger representative tissue sections from the tumor, since the diagnosis relies on the amount of mitoses found in selected areas of the tumor.

Occasionally interposed vessels between the transducer and the lesion may prevent a biopsy (Fig. 20.1). Unfortunately, this is often the case in patients with lesions in the liver hilum. Gastric lesions are among the most difficult to biopsy, and insuffi-

---

* see reference list on pp. 171 ff.

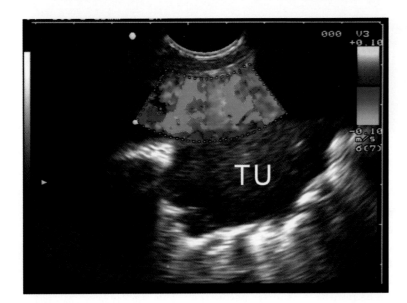

Fig. 20.1. Limitations of EUS guided biopsy. A vessel is outlined by color Doppler imaging in front of a hypoechoic lesion (*TU*), preventing biopsy.

cient material is collected in a high percentage of these cases. This is due, in part, to the tendency of the elastic gastric wall to move in conjunction with the to-and-fro needle movement. Firm lesions may be difficult to penetrate with the needle tip, and it may be necessary to perform the initial penetration with a sudden forceful movement of the needle. This situation arises routinely in pancreatic tumors, which often contain a large amount of fibrotic tissue.

In conclusion, EUS-FNA is an important addition to endosonography and has expanded the clinical role of EUS. The possibility of obtaining cytological and histological samples from lesions visualized by EUS has significantly changed the indications for patient referral to our hospital. We now perform EUS-FNA in about 40% of all EUS examinations.

The advantage of the high frequency, high resolution transducers used for endosonography combined with the ability to biopsy lesions that are difficult to visualize and diagnose with other imaging modalities makes EUS-FNA a valuable diagnostic tool.

PART 5

Therapy

CHAPTER 21

Interventional Therapeutic Endosonography: Current Status

H. Seifert

History, Introduction

Interventional Endosonography (EUS) is the logical consequence of the combination of interventional endoscopy and interventional ultrasound. The idea of tissue sampling or minimally invasive interventions resulted from insights gained through these techniques.

Since the early 1970s, the domain of interventional ultrasonography has been diagnostic and therapeutic puncture or drainage of almost any region of the human body. Numerous types of needles have been developed, and ultrasound units have reached a technical level in which their images match those obtained by the most advanced radiological techniques. Data regarding efficacy and complication rates of sonographic interventions are based on a large numbers of patients. Some 25 years ago, endoscopic interventions were pioneered not only by the first papillotomies, but also by the puncture of cystic lesions (Rogers, Cicurel et al. 1975; Cremer, Deviere et al. 1989; Sahel 1990).

Combining both the sonographic and the endoscopic approach brought the endocopist's eye into a formerly unknown territory: the organs adjacent to the upper and lower gastrointestinal tract. Endosonography allowed insights into "black boxes" such as the mediastinum around the esophagus, the pancreatic tail, or the peripapillary region. Soon after echoendoscopes became available, EUS guided FNA was attempted. The advantage of performing FNA with the transducer very close to the target, however, was counterbalanced by technical difficulties. It was much harder to stabilize the transducer with the needle tip and the target in the visual field than with conventional ultrasound, and there was no standard equipment available such as long needles or catheters. Although in the meantime, different needle types have been established for EUS guided aspiration cytology, EUS guided FNA remains technically demanding. For puncture and drainage of cysts, technical details are still in the process of development.

Instruments

Radial and Mechanical Scanners

Radial scanners create an 360°-sonographic image comparable to a disc mounted onto the tip of an endoscope. This is ideal for anatomical orientation, but not suitable to control endoscopic interventions. Because a needle introduced through the working channel would cut through the sonographic plane of a radial scanner at precisely one point, the needle tract would virtually be out of endosonographic control. Nevertheless, FNA guided by radially scanning EUS has been attempted.

In 1995, a mechanical 7.5 MHz scanner was introduced for EUS guided punctures (Olympus GF-UMP 30). This instrument uses a mirror to direct the ultrasound beam of a rotating crystal into a forward 250° imaging plane. It has a 2.8 mm working channel and allows guided punctures using the same ultrasound unit as in diagnostic EUS with mechanical radial scanners. The theoretical advantage of the large imaging sector, however, is counterbalanced by a slightly reduced image quality.

Electronical Longitudinal Scanners

Curved linear array electronical scanners with the ultrasound transducer in a longitudinal plane suitable to visualize most of the needle tract have been developed. With these instruments anatomical orientation was more difficult than with radial scanners, but EUS guided FNA became feasible for the first time. While several prototype instrument images were suboptimal, in the early 1990s the Pentax FG 32UVA became the standard longitudinal EUS-scanner. With a frequency of 7.5 MHz, reliable quality of the endoscope, a working channel of 2.0 mm, and a sonographic image quality derived from and equal to standard conventional ultrasound, this instrument led to the first large series of EUS guided diagnostic punctures. Fine needle aspiration cytologies (FNAC) were obtained from lesions formerly difficult to reach (see chapter VI). Pancreatic pseudocysts, even without bulging of the gastric or duodenal wall, were transmurally punctured and drained under direct EUS-control.

While linear EUS improved the safety of these puncture procedures, their technical execution was often complicated because of the small working channels of the available instruments. In FNAC, the recently developed needles with a durable and relatively stiff protective sheath were hard to maneuver. Direct drainage was impossible because stents of sufficient size could not be passed through the biopsy channel. As a consequence, larger instruments were developed. First, the FG 36UX (Hitachi/Pentax) with a 2.4 mm working channel was introduced, followed by the GF UC 30 P with a 2.8 mm working channel (Olympus) and the FG 38UX (Hitachi/Pentax) with a 3.2 mm working channel.

Indications and Applications: Drainage of Abscesses and Pseudocysts

Transmural drainage of perigastric and periduodenal cystic lesions is the most important indication of therapeutic interventional EUS. It will be described here in detail. Other applications, such as EUS guided local instillation of anesthetics and other agents are less well established and will be dealt with in the following chapter.

Drainage of Abscesses and Pseudocysts

Endoscopic therapy of pancreatic pseudocysts has been established during recent years. For guidance of transmural punctures and drainages, endoscopic ultrasound (EUS) has been employed to improve the safety of these procedures (Grimm, Binmoeller et al. 1992; Binmoeller, Seifert et al. 1995). Recently, we have performed all transmural drainages under EUS-control in order to treat difficult to reach cysts and to minimize the risk of bleeding complications (Fig. 21.1). However, the available EUS-endoscopes did not permit the passage of catheters or stents sufficiently large for abscess drainage. Therefore, EUS guided FNA had to be followed by the placement of a guide wire into the target cavity. Subsequently, the echoendoscope was exchanged over the wire for a large-channel instrument and stent in-

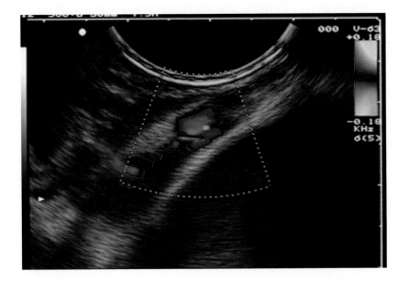

Fig. 21.1. Gastric position of the ultrasonic transducer (Pentax FG 38UX, 7.5 MHz). Proximal is *left*. Between the gastric wall and the large, anechoic pseudocyst (*lower right*), a large interposed artery is visualized, which prohibits puncture at this site.

sertion was performed without EUS-control. This procedure was technically demanding, time consuming, and sometimes frustrating when the wire slipped out during the exchange of the instruments.

Using the longitudinal scanning echoendoscope (FG 38UX with a 3.2 mm working channel), EUS guided punctures immediately followed by the insertion of 7, 8, or 8.5F stents became possible. Different needle-stent devices for transmural one-step puncture and drainage of cystic lesions adjacent to the gastric or duodenal wall were developed. Indications for endoscopic therapy and their techniques will now be discussed.

Indications

Most cystic lesions treated by endoscopical transmural drainage are pancreatic pseudocysts due to chronic or, less commonly, acute pancreatitis. However, the therapeutic options described below and their indications apply to almost any pathological fluid collection within the reach of the echoendoscope. Because there is neither a good systematic definition of intraabdominal cysts (pancreatic pseudocysts, postacute fluid collections, infected necrosis, abscesses, with and without connection to the pancreatic duct, with or without a "wall" etc.) nor any reliable criteria to predict their natural development and risk of complications (will they grow, rupture, bleed, lead to sepsis, or resolve spontaneously?), a pragmatic approach appears reasonable. From here on, pseudocysts and other cystic lesions will be called "cysts". Treatment decisions can be based primarily on symptoms. Asymptomatic cysts should be treated only when a malignancy is suspected (diagnostic puncture), or when they are infected (prevention of septic complications). Pain and biliary, gastric or duodenal obstruction are symptoms justifying treatment. In most cases, an observation period of 4-6 weeks seems justified because spontaneous resolution has been reported for cysts of any size.

Surgery, percutaneous drainage, and therapeutic endoscopy offer a variety of treatment options that can be tailored according to the needs of individual patients.

If accessible, cysts are preferentially treated by endoscopic drainage at our institution. This approach has the advantages of minimizing invasiveness, reducing patient discomfort, shortening the needle tract used and lowering complication rates. More aggressive surgical approaches are not an alternative strategy, but a second line therapy when endoscopic therapy fails. Surgical therapy of cysts, comprising various techniques, is principally based on drainage via pancreatico- or cysto-jejunostomy. None of these procedures, which usually require a Roux-en-Y anastomosis, are always successful or without complications. Postoperative morbidity is higher than in interventional endoscopy. Nevertheless, interventional endoscopic therapy of cystic lesions essentially is minimally invasive surgery. It should only be carried out with adequate surgical backup.

Pre-procedure imaging by abdominal ultrasound, CT, or occasionally additional imaging techniques such as miniprobe-EUS is obligatory.

Technical Procedures

Transpapillary drainage can be performed if the pseudocyst communicates with the pancreatic duct and is easily accessible via transpapillary cannulation. Whether cases with small fistulas of the pancreatic duct should be stabilized by a pancreatic prosthesis and cystic drainage performed transmurally, rather than dilating the fistular tract by transpapillary techniques and providing transfistular drainage is not clear and cannot be answered based on published studies. In cases of cysts that compress the duodenum or the pancreatic duct and impede pancreatography, we prefer transmural drainage as a first therapeutic step. Sometimes in a second session, after resolution of the cyst, the previously distorted anatomy is easily clarified by EUS and ERCP.

In cases with obvious bulging of the intestinal wall, a short puncture distance, and no interposed vessels seen by radial-scanning EUS, punctures can be carried out under endoscopic control only, if there is no longitudinally scanning echoendoscope available. If the anatomy is more complicated (no bulging, interposed vessels, small cysts, or a long puncture distance), we consider EUS guided puncture obligatory.

Technical details of puncture and drainage, depending on the echoendoscope used, can either be classified a as a two-step or a one-step method

(Seifert, Dietrich et al. 1999/2000). In the latter, puncture and drainage are carried out with one echoendoscope. In the two-step method, EUS guided puncture is followed by drainage using a large-channel endoscope. Although there is no standardized technique, the following description of our approach may serve as a guideline.

Cysts are localized and the optimal site for puncture established. Sonographic coupling is obtained by minimizing intraluminal air and by direct contact of the transducer to the intestinal wall. This sometimes requires 100 ml of water filling. No balloon insufflation is used. All punctures are carried out under direct endosonographic control without endoscopic guidance during the intervention. Fluoroscopy is used in all cases for documentation, and as an additional control to ensure the correct placement of the needle and the guidewire within the cyst.

The Two-Step Technique

If echoendoscopes with narrow working channels (2.0 mm) have to be used, FNA can be performed with a needle knife or in our preference a 0.7 mm full length steel needle (EchoTip, Wilson-Cook Medical, Winston-Salem, N.C., USA; GIP, Grassau, Germany). After a 5 F-plastic catheter is passed over the needle, the cystic lumen is reached with a 0.035″ guide wire. Alternatively, a 0.018″ steel wire can be introduced directly through needle. For the second step, the echoendoscope is now exchanged over the guide wire for a therapeutic large-channel (3.7 or 4.2 mm) endoscope. A gastroscope or a duodenoscope is used according to the individual anatomy. Finally, a 10 F Teflon-stent is inserted for drainage, analogous to endoscopic biliary drainage.

The One-Step Technique

For one-step puncture-drainage procedures, we use needles that are made of stainless steel, have a 1 mm outer diameter, are 160 cm in length, have a sharpened beveled tip, and are equipped with a blunted stylet (Grosse, Daldorf, Germany). The needle is loaded with a 7 F Teflon pusher and a modified 6 cm long 7 F Teflon stent (Wilson-Cook, Winston-Salem, N.C., USA) with two sideholes and 4 flaps in order to prevent dislocation.

Once the echoendoscope is placed in a stable position, the needle is advanced until it causes a slight impression on the intestinal wall at the desired spot. The needle tip, after it is sharpened by retracting the stylet about one centimeter, is anchored within the gastric or duodenal wall. At this point, a final correction of the echoendoscope's position is often necessary to optimize targeting while keeping the needle in the sonographic plane. After the needle tip is advanced into the cystic lumen with a firm push, the stylet is withdrawn and about 10 ml of aspirate is obtained from the cyst for diagnostic testing. A few milliliters of diluted contrast medium, injected through the needle, gives endosonographic (Fig. 21.2) and fluoroscopic (Fig. 21.3) proof of the correct intracystic position of the needle. In large cysts, this is followed by advancing the needle with the stent into its final position. Once the prosthesis

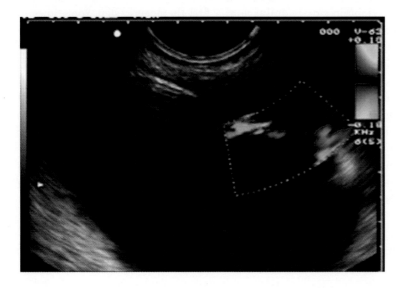

Fig. 21.2. The needle is inside the lumen of a large pseudocyst. Fluid injection leads to a water jet visible on color Doppler confirming correct position of the needle tip. Note the gastric position of the ultrasound transducer. (Hitachi FG 38UX, 7.5 MHz)

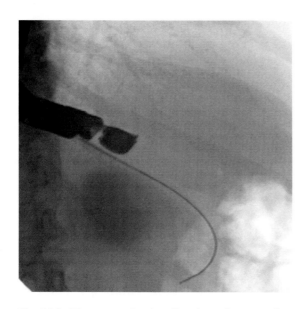

Fig. 21.3. Fluoroscopic visualization of FNA. After injection of a small amount of diluted contrast agent, a stainless steel guide wire is introduced through the needle to secure its position inside the cystic lumen.

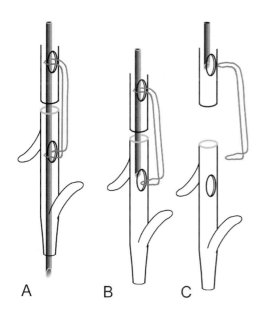

Fig. 21.4. Schematic drawing of the needle-and-stent device for one-step puncture-drainage procedures. *A*) The assembly consisting of the needle and the 7-F pusher with the 7-F stent connected by the thread. The stylet was withdrawn previously. *B*) after correct positioning, the needle is carefully retracted with the pusher holding the stent in place. The stent is then released. *C*) The pusher and needle are then withdrawn.

is placed as desired, the needle and the pusher are withdrawn. The needle and the stent can be readily differentiated endosonographically. If we feel that the needle tip could extend beyond the back of the cyst or that the position is not stable, a 0.018 inch steel guide wire with a flexible tip (Access, Cook, Mönchengladbach, Germany) is passed through the needle into the cyst. Coated wires should be avoided because of the risk of damaging them through the sharp needle. In small cysts, saline injection after a diagnostic aspiration has proven useful in preventing collapse of the lumen and in facilitating stent placement.

In order to allow optimal positioning of the stent, a simple but effective construction is implemented into the needle device (Fig. 21.4). An additional side hole is cut 5 mm from the distal end of the pusher catheter, with another one 5 mm off the proximal end of the prosthesis. The latter is attached to the pusher by a loop of surgical suture material (Prolene 3/0, Ethicon, Norderstedt, Germany) that goes into both holes and around the needle as shown. With this device the prosthesis is not released before it is correctly placed and the fixation-loop set free by withdrawing the needle.

After successful drainage, the cyst almost always collapses and often completely resolves within a few days. For lasting success and low recurrence rates, some basic principles should be taken into account. The position of the stent and its functioning should be controlled and documented immediately after the procedure (Fig. 21.5). The first examination should be by abdominal ultrasound on the day following the intervention. Endoscopic evaluation should be scheduled within the first week. It should check the stent position and patency, and if necessary, insert a larger stent or even dilate the transmural fenestration and insert a 7 F-nasocystic catheter. This is very effective, especially in cysts containing viscous debris or putrid material (Fig. 21.6). Ideally a 7 F-nasocystic catheter is used for flushing while the 10 F-stent or a wide fenestration (or both) provide drainage into the gastric or duodenal lumen. In complicated and infected cysts, flushing should be done at least 3 times daily with a daily volume of at least 1000 ml. We have used saline or Ringer's solution up to around 1500 ml/d or until diarrhea resulted. With this approach, even cysts containing solid necrosis can be cleaned completely. In individual cases, we have used 10 F-catheters attached to

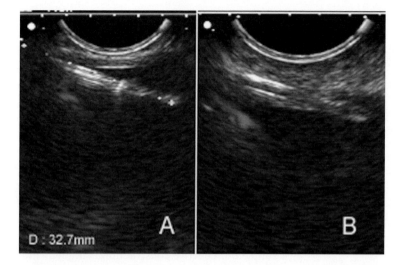

Fig. 21.5. The desired position of the 7-F stent with the needle tip (*A*), and after withdrawing the needle (*B*), is clearly visualized on EUS. (Pentax FG 38UX, 7.5 MHz)

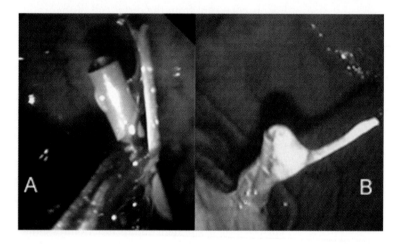

Fig. 21.6. Endoscopic images after transgastric EUS guided drainage. (*A*) Flow of clear cystic contents immediately after a one-step drainage procedure. The released connecting thread is seen. (*B*) A 7-F stent immediately after the procedure with putrid material emptying from an infected cyst. Both lesions resolved completely after an exchange of stents.

a strong suction pump to extract lumps of necrosis through the transmural channel.

Outcome

Cystic lesions within the reach of EUS can be successfully punctured and drained at least 90% of the time. The major complication is bleeding, which can be minimized by EUS with color Doppler (Fig. 21.1). The bleeding rate should be less than 5%. One death attributable to the procedure has been reported. Recurrence rates range from 6 to 18% with follow up as long as 7 years. Lasting success in terms of clinical outcome is hard to measure because of the difficulty in the treatment of chronic pancreatitis. In this context, it must be emphasized that endoscopic

treatment of pancreatic pseudocysts only makes sense as part of a comprehensive therapeutic strategy comprising transpapillary stenting, dilation of strictures, stone extraction and, if necessary, lithotripsy.

Endoscopic drainage provides a minimally invasive approach to pseudocyst management, with success and recurrence rates at least equal to those of open surgery but with lower morbidity and mortality rates. It should be considered as the treatment of choice for cystic abdominal lesions.

Differentiation of neoplastic from benign cystic lesions is most important and this can be accomplished based on patient history, cystic morphology, and with EUS guided FNA providing diagnostic specimens for cytopathology, histopathology, and aspirate from the cystic lumen for determination of tumor markers.

Y. K. Chen · K. J. Chang

CHAPTER 22
Interventional Therapeutic Endosonography: Future Perspectives

Background

Since endoscopic ultrasound (EUS) was introduced more than 15 years ago, this modality has become established as a highly accurate means of staging gastrointestinal and pancreatic malignancies. Recent technological advancements have overcome some of the initial limitations of EUS and introduced a growing list of potential therapeutic applications. Thus, EUS is beginning to find a niche in the armamentarium of minimally-invasive interventional techniques.

EUS is now recognized as the single best modality for the detection of pancreatic tumors with a reported sensitivity of over 95% (Roesch et al. 1992). In addition, EUS is now established as the best modality for local staging of esophageal, gastric and rectal cancer with a T stage accuracy of approximately 90% (Akahoshi et al. 1991; Boyce et al. 1992; Rice et al. 1992). Despite this, EUS has not gained widespread acceptance in clinical practice, in part because EUS has limited specificity if used purely as an imaging modality, particularly when it comes to distinguishing metastatic lymph nodes from benign inflammatory nodes. The accuracy of EUS nodal staging for all gastrointestinal malignancies is approximately 80% (Grimm et al. 1992). This accuracy is further reduced in the subgroup of patients with less advanced T-stage tumors in whom the prevalence of local metastases is low. Thus, the test is highly sensitive but lacks specificity. Likewise, EUS cannot reliably distinguish pancreatic cancer from focal pancreatitis. The specificity of EUS for pancreatic cancer has been reported to be only 76% (Roesch et al. 1991). Recent reports suggest that EUS guided FNA and other interventional applications of EUS will increase the diagnostic capabilities of EUS, allow for minimally invasive delivery of therapeutic agents, and demonstrate the cost-effectiveness of this technology.

EUS Guided FNA

The radial scanning echoendoscope does not permit EUS guided FNA because the aspiration needle is seen only in cross section; the endosonographer cannot safely advance the tip of the needle into the target lesion under direct ultrasound guidance. The first echoendoscope with an electronic sector scanner oriented along the long axis of the scope (FG-32UA) was introduced by Pentax/Hitachi seven years ago. With this orientation, an aspiration needle could be inserted through the operating channel and the entire needle visualized with real-time ultrasound. This innovation was a major breakthrough because it made the technique of EUS guided FNA technically feasible. The EUS linear array orientation and technique of EUS guided FNA are presented elsewhere in this textbook and in previous reviews. Multiple reports of EUS guided FNA have demonstrated its technical feasibility, relative safety, and high cytologic yield.

Interventional EUS

In the same way that fluoroscopy, transcutaneous ultrasound, and CT are used by the radiologist to assist with various therapeutic interventions, recent developments in EUS technology have propelled EUS from a purely diagnostic tool to become a therapeutic instrument in the hands of the endosonographer. The evolving clinical applications of EUS parallel the development of endoscopic retrograde cholangiopancreatography (ERCP), albeit in a more accelerated timeline. By progressing from a purely imaging modality (EUS alone), to a modality that provides a tissue diagnosis (EUS guided FNA), to a modality that provides therapy (interventional EUS), it is anticipated that the clinical and economic impact of EUS will continue to increase.

Recent reports have described the technique of fine needle injection of therapeutic agents and other interventional EUS applications. Novel therapeutic applications of EUS guided FNI include celiac plexus neurolysis (Wiersema and Wiersema, 1996) and injection of botulinum toxin (Hoffman et al. 1996) and anti-tumor agents (Chang et al. 1998). In addition, the next generation of therapeutic echoendoscopes will have a larger operating channel, making it easier to perform combined diagnostic/interventional procedures with the same instrument.

EUS Guided FNI

Celiac Nerve Block

Neurolytic therapy for chronic abdominal pain due to pancreatic cancer or chronic pancreatitis has traditonally relied upon surgical, fluoroscopic and CT-guidance to locate and access the celiac ganglion nerve plexus. Intraoperatively, the celiac artery is identified and its surrounding area injected with a neurolytic agent, usually ethyl alcohol or bupivacaine. Injections into the celiac trunk can also be accomplished using fluoroscopy to guide the needle into the area anterolateral to the T12 spine and adjacent to the lateral aspect of the aorta, via a posterior percutaneous approach. An anterior approach is commonly preferred with CT guidance. Compared with fluoroscopy, the CT guided technique is more precise and has a higher success rate, approaching 70-90%.

More recently, EUS has been shown to be suitable for guiding injections of neurolytic agents into the celiac plexus. Using a linear array echoendoscope (Pentax Precision Instruments, Orangeburg, NY; Olympus Corporation, Melville, NY), the trunk of the celiac artery is easily identified as it branches off from the abdominal aorta. A 22 gauge needle (GIP/Mediglobe, Tempe, AZ; Olympus Corporation, Melville, NY; Wilson-Cook Medical, Winston-Salem, NC) is passed through the operating channel and, under real-time ultrasound guidance, advanced

through the gastric wall into the area surrounding the celiac trunk. Injection of bupivacaine (0.25%) and ethyl alcohol (98%) can then be performed.

The safety and efficacy of EUS guided celiac nerve block in 25 patients with pancreatic carcinoma and five patients with intra-abdominal metastases has been reported recently (Wiersema and Wiersema, 1996). This study showed that the pain score as measured by a visual analog scale is significantly lower at 2, 4, 8, and 12 weeks when compared with baseline. During follow-up, 82% to 91% of patients required the same or a lower dose of pain-medication and 79% to 88% of patients had persistent improvement in their pain score. The complications of EUS guided celiac nerve block were minor and consisted of transient diarrhea in four patients.

Unfortunately when used to treat patients with chronic pain due to chronic pancreatitis, EUS guided celiac nerve block does not appear to produce equivalent benefits. Harada et al. compared the efficacy of EUS guided blockade in nine patients with intractable abdominal pain secondary to chronic pancreatitis with 58 patients with intra-abdominal malignancy (Harada et al. 1997). The two patient groups had similar initial pain scores. During post-treatment follow-up, patients with malignancy had a significantly lower pain score compared with their baseline value ($P < 0.001$), whereas, patients with chronic pancreatitis did not experience any pain relief. Using the Kaplan-Meier estimate, the median duration of efficacious pain control for malignant disease was 20 weeks compared with only two weeks for patients with chronic pancreatitis ($P = 0.008$). The authors reported minor complications including transient diarrhea and increased pain. (Gress et al.) performed EUS guided celiac nerve block in 80 patients with chronic pancreatitis (Gress et al. 1997). The investigators injected a mixture containing 20 ml of bupivacaine 0.25% and 80 mg of triamcinolone (6 ml). Fifty-five percent of patients reported a 50% or more decrease in their global pain score at seven days. Twenty-five percent of patients reported a persistent benefit beyond 12 weeks, but only ten percent still had a benefit at 24 weeks. There were two major complications (2.5%): a peripancreatic abscess that was diagnosed five days after the procedure and a bleeding celiac artery due to an ethanol-induced pseudoaneurysm.

Although there are no randomized studies, EUS guided celiac nerve block for pancreatic cancer patients appears to be as effective as the more traditional approaches, and the technique is associated with a comparable low complication rate. One advantage of EUS guided celiac nerve block is that during EUS staging of patients with pancreatic cancer, those patients who are found to have unresectable disease and significant pain may immediately be offered EUS guided celiac block, thus avoiding the cost and inconvenience of a second procedure. The efficacy of EUS guided celiac nerve block for patients with chronic pancreatitis appears limited.

Injection of Anti-tumor Agents

A natural extension of EUS guided fine needle injection (FNI) is to use it to deliver chemotherapeutic or biological agents directly into tumors. We have recently conducted a Phase I clinical trial employing the new technique of EUS guided injection for delivering local immunotherapy in patients with advanced pancreatic cancer (Chang et al. 1998). Eight patients with unresectable adenocarcinoma of the pancreas (stage II-4, stage III-3, stage IV-1) were enrolled. Cytoimplants were delivered locally into the tumor by a single EUS guided FNI in escalating doses of 3, 6 or 9 billion cells. There were two partial responders and one minor responder, with a median survival of 13 months. No bone marrow, hemorrhagic, infectious, renal, cardiac or pulmonary toxicities were encountered. Three patients developed a transient grade 3 toxicity, and three patients had transient hyperbilirubinemia which resolved with biliary stent exchange. Seven of the eight patients experienced a low grade fever which responded to acetaminophen; all resolved within four weeks. There were no procedure-related complications. Our data suggests that local immunotherapy is technically feasible and safe, and holds significant promise for wider clinical application. An expanded multicenter study is currently in progress.

Botulinum Toxin Injection

Another example of interventional EUS is EUS guided injection of botulinum toxin in patients with achalasia. Hoffman et al. treated 7 patients with EUS guided injection of botulinum toxin into the lower esophageal sphincter, 20 units in each of 4 quadrants.

Six of the 7 patients had no dysphagia at a mean follow-up of 6.5 months (Hoffman et al. 1996). Whether EUS guided injection improves the therapeutic outcome is uncertain, and there is a need for further evaluation in a prospective randomized fashion. Similarly, using EUS to guide the injections of botulinum toxin or other agents into the anal sphincter for management of proctalgia fugax, the painful levator syndrome, and anal fissures awaits future investigation.

EUS Guided Cholangiopancreatography

EUS guided transduodenal cholangiography and EUS guided transgastric pancreatography have been described. Clinical situations where EUS guided cholangiography will be a useful alternative include failed transpapillary cholangiography, complete obstruction of the common bile duct, pyloric or duodenal stenosis, and any altered UGI anatomy precluding endoscopic access to the papilla of Vater. Likewise, in patients with an inaccesible or completely obstructed main pancreatic duct secondary to any etiology, EUS guided transgastric pancreatography can provide additional information regarding both the pancreatic parenchyma and the ductal system proximal to the obstruction, which may aid the surgeon in planning the most appropriate surgical approach.

Other Interventional EUS Applications

Pancreatic Pseudocyst Drainage

EUS may have a role in both the evaluation and treatment of pancreatic cysts. Prior to performing endoscopic cyst-enterostomy, EUS guided FNA may help to localize the cyst and differentiate pancreatic pseudocysts from other types of cysts and cyst neoplasms. Dancour et al. evaluated 19 patients with 23 pancreatic cysts by using EUS guided FNA (Dancour et al. 1996). The cyst fluid was analyzed for cytology (n=23), bacteriology (n=1), pancreatic enzymes, and tumor markers (CEA, CA 19-9) (n=13). EUS guided FNA established the correct diagnosis in 83% of patients. Once the diagnosis of a pseudocyst has been established, EUS may be helpful to determine the suitability of endoscopic cyst drainage, to direct cyst-puncture, to measure the cyst and the distance for transmural puncture, and to place a guidewire and plastic stent(s) into the pseudocyst. Endosonographic visualization of anatomic details, especially submucosal vessels and gastric varices, lowers the risk of bleeding and perforation. Even cyst drainage in anatomically difficult positions can be attempted under direct EUS control. Binmoeller et al. performed EUS guided transgastric (*n*=8) or transduodenal (*n*=1) drainage procedures in 9 patients with symptomatic pseudocysts (Binmoeller and Soehendra, 1995). At endoscopy, two patients did not have visible bulging of the gastric wall. Cyst puncture and drainage was successful in all patients. Stent clogging resulted in pseudocyst infection in 3 patients, which was successfully treated with stent exchange and cyst irrigation. During a follow-up period of 3-12 months, serial abdominal sonography showed complete disappearance of pseudocysts in 5 patients, and marked reduction of the size of the cysts in four patients. Self-limited bleeding occurred in one patient during cyst puncture.

Common Bile Duct Stones

EUS can be used as an adjunct to ERCP in the detection of common bile duct stones. Three published series of over 200 patients have shown that EUS has a sensitivity of 88-97% and a specificity of 97-100% for detecting choledocholithiasis (Edmundowicz 1995). Thus, there may be a clinical role for EUS in the evaluation of patients suspected to have choledocholithiasis. However, the use of EUS may be limited to the evaluation of patients with a moderate probability of choledocholithiasis. Used in this context, ERCP can be performed selectively for patients who are found to have bile duct stones on EUS. Patients who are found to have stones on transcutaneous ultrasound and patients who have a high clinical probability of having choledocholithiasis may be treated with ERCP and subsequently cholecystectomy. Those with a low probability may be referred directly for a cholecystectomy. This algorithm has the potential of decreasing the number of ERCP-related complications. A recent cost-analysis study suggests that this algorithm could be cost-effective (Erickson and Chang, 1996). Whether EUS has a role in the evaluation of patients with severe acute gallstone pancreatitis is unclear and studies have been initiated to address this issue.

EUS-Assisted Endoscopic Mucosal Resection

Endoscopy and barium studies cannot accurately diagnose submucosal gastrointestinal tract lesions. EUS is useful for localizing tumors within the gastrointestinal wall, differentiating submucosal tumors from vascular structures and extrinsic organs, and assessing their size and depth of invasion. However, echosonographic imaging criteria alone may not reliably distinguish between benign and malignant submucosal lesions, and submucosal lesions are not histologically accessible by routine endoscopic mucosal biopsies. Because of these limitations, endoscopic mucosal resection (EMR) is gaining increasing acceptance as a management alternative for deep mucosal and submucosal lesions. Otherwise known as strip biopsy, EMR decreases the need for follow-up endoscopy or EUS, either by removing the entire lesion or by confirming its benign histology. Furthermore, EMR for early gastric cancer and other gastrointestinal malignancies has been widely accepted as a standard treatment in Japan due to its minimal invasiveness. To increase the safety of EMR, some investigators perform submucosal injections of physiologic saline, epinephrine 1:10,000, Dextrose 50% solution, or banding prior to EMR, in order to minimize the risk of perforation and inadvertent resection of the deep muscle layer. In addition, EUS can be used to confirm submucosal bleb injection or band location prior to EMR. Preliminary reports suggest that EUS-assisted EMR is a safe technique for obtaining a deep tissue diagnosis or removing selected submucosal tumors in the GI-tract (Chen et al. 1999; Kawamoto et al. 1997).

"Intensive" Variceal Ligation

The majority of esophageal variceal eradication therapy is directed at the distal 5 cm of the esophagus, where most of the variceal bleeding events occur. Using cadaveric specimens, Vianna et al. described four distinct anatomic zones of venous drainage all predominantly localized within the esophageal mucosal folds: gastric, palisade, perforating and truncal (Vianna et al. 1987). Nagamine et al. speculated that the palisade and perforating zones of the venous drainage were critical to the formation of varices and their rupture and should therefore be the target of EUS-assisted, modified, or "intensive" band ligation (Nagamine et al. 1998). Because the standard echoendoscope causes compression deformity of the varices in question (Nagamine et al.) used a transendoscopic 15-mHz or 20 mHz radial scanning ultrasound miniprobe and a 7.5-mHz electronic linear array device for color Doppler (CD) imaging in order to monitor the hemodynamics of varices before and after endoscopic variceal ligation. In a series of 38 patients undergoing this EUS-CD assisted intensive banding method, the investigators reported that recurrence of varices occurred after a mean of 18 months, which compares favorably with the average recurrence at 6 months previously reported with conventional band ligation. Endoscopic ultrasound localization of varices, identification of perforating veins, and monitoring of variceal occlusion with transendoscopically placed miniprobes and EUS-CD are novel applications of EUS technology. However, prospective randomized studies and a longer duration of follow-up are needed to evaluate both the long-term effectiveness of EUS-assisted modified band ligation and the clinical usefulness of EUS-CD assisted modified band ligation.

Future Developments in Interventional EUS

The next generation of therapeutic echoendoscopes now being field-tested are equipped with a large (3.7 mm) operating channel which can accommodate bigger accessories and stent sizes. Future echoendoscope refinements will include a reduction in the size and length of the transducer head, which should make it easier to maneuver the scope tip, localize the papilla of Vater, and position the accessories to perform endoscopic sphincterotomy, stone extraction, stent placement and other interventional procedures without having to switch endoscopes. In cases of failed transpapillary cannulation, pre-cut sphincterotomy can be limited to those patients who are found to have definite biliary pathology at EUS that justifies the risks of pre-cut sphincterotomy, which is then performed by using the same therapeutic echoendoscope. Those patients without EUS abnormalities could still have an EUS guided cholangiography during the same procedure.

Preliminary studies using a pig model suggest that it may be technically feasible to perform EUS guided hepaticogastrostomy for palliation of malignant obstructive jaundice (Sahai et al. 1998). A chronic bilio-gastric fistula could result after stent removal thereby obviating the need for periodic stent exchanges. Similarly, in selected patients who fail transpapillary cannulation of an obstructed bile duct, it may be possible to access the bile duct via an EUS guided transgastric or transduodenal puncture proximal to the level of obstruction, followed by antegrade placement of an exchange guidewire through the papilla, thus avoiding a combined percutaneous-endoscopic procedure.

It can be anticipated in the future that various fine needle or wire-type ablation devices will be available, which may be positioned with real time endosonographic guidance into a benign or malignant target lesion, for delivery of thermal, electrical, ultrasonic or cryotherapy (freeze probe) treatments without causing unintended injury to the gut wall and other surrounding tissues along the path of the delivery device.

Conclusions

EUS is both a diagnostic and therapeutic modality and holds significant promise for widespread clinical use. The emergence of EUS guided FNA and EUS guided FNI has opened the door for multiple interventional applications. These new and evolving applications of EUS will increase the cost-effectiveness of EUS in the diagnosis and treatment of gastrointestinal and pancreatic diseases.

Appendix

References

Akahoshi K, Misawa T, Fujishima H et al (1991) Preoperative evaluation of gastric cancer by endoscopic ultrasound. Gut 32:479–482

Anonymous (1993) Clinical applications of endoscopic ultrasonography in gastroenterology – state of the art 1993. Results of a consensus conference, Orlando, Florida, 19 January 1993. Endoscopy 25(5):358–366

Anonymous (1995) EUS-guided biopsy of pancreatic lesions suspected of malignancy. A multicentre study. Acta Endosc 25:465–471

Anonymous (1996) Guidelines of the European Society of Gastrointestinal Endoscopy (ESGE) Endoscopic ultrasonography. I. Technique and upper gastrointestinal tract. European Endosonography Club. Endoscopy 28(5):474–476

Bibra H, Becher H, Firschke C et al (1993) Enhancement of mitral regurgitation and normal left arterial color Doppler flow signals with peripheral venous injection of a saccharide-based contrast agent. J Am Coll Cardiol 22:521–528

Binmoeller KF, Jabusch HC, Seifert H, Soehendra N (1997) Endosonography-guided fine-needle biopsy of indurated pancreatic lesions using an automated biopsy device. Endoscopy 29:384–388

Binmoeller KF, Soehendra N (1995) Endoscopic ultrasonography in the diagnosis and treatment of pancreatic pseudocysts. Gastrointest Endosc Clin N Am 5:805–816

Binmoeller KF, Seifert H et al (1995) Transpapillary and transmural drainage of pancreatic pseudocysts. Gastrointestinal Endoscopy 42(3):219–224

Boyce GA, Sivak MV Jr, Lavery IC et al (1992) Endoscopic ultrasound in the pre-operative staging of rectal carcinoma. Gastrointest Endosc 38:468–471

Burtin P, Palazzo L, Canard JM, Person B, Oberti F, Boyer J (1997) Diagnostic strategies for extrahepatic cholestasis of indefinite origin: endoscopic ultrasonography or retrograde cholangiography? Results of a prospective study. Endoscopy 29(5):349–355

Caletti G, Devière J, Fockens P, Lees WR, Mortensen B, Odegaard S, Rösch T, Souquet JS, Vilmann P (1996) Guidelines of the European Society of Gastrointestinal Endoscopy (ESGE). II. retroperitoneum and large bowel, training. The European Endosonography Club Working Party. Endoscopy 28(7):626–628

Caletti G, Fusaroli P, Bocus P (1998) Endoscopic ultrasonography. Digestion 59(5):509–529

Canto MI, Chak A, Stellato T, Sivak MV Jr (1998) Endoscopic ultrasonography versus cholangiography for the diagnosis of choledocholithiasis. Gastrointest Endosc 47(6):439–448

Chang K, Nguyen P, Erickson RA, Durbin TE, Katz KD (1997) The clinical utility of endoscopic ultrasound guided aspiration in the diagnosis and staging of pancreatic carcinoma. Gastrointest Endosc 45:387–393

Chang K, Nguyen P, Thompson J et al (1998) Phase I Clinical Trial of Allogeneic Mixed Lymphocyte Culture (cytoimplant) delivered by endoscopic ultrasound (EUS)-guided fine needle injection (FNI) in patients with advanced pancreatic carcinoma. Gastrointest Endosc 47:AB144

Chang KJ, Katz KD, Durbin ED et al (1994) Endoscopic ultrasound-guided fine-needle aspiration. Gastrointest Endosc 40:694–699

Chen YK, Nguyen P, Lin F, Tran PN, Chang KJ (1999) Endoscopic-ultrasound (EUS) assisted endoscopic mucosal resection (EMR) of deep GI mucosal and submucosal lesions. Gastrointest Endosc (in press)

Cremer M, Deviere J et al (1989) Endoscopic management of cysts and pseudocysts in chronic pancreatitis: long-term follow-up after 7 years of experience. Gastrointestinal Endoscopy 35(1):1–9

Crouse LJ, Cheirif J, Hanly DE, Kisslo JA, Labovitz AJ, Raichelen JS (1993) Opacification and border delineation improvement in patients with suboptimal endocardial border definition in routine echocardiography: results of phase III Albunex multicenter trial. J Am Coll Cardiol 22:1494–1500

Dancour A, Sosa Valencia L, Molas G et al (1996) Fine-needle aspiration (FNA) during sectorial endosonography (ES) is useful for the etiological diagnosis of pancreatic cysts. Gastroenterology 110:A385

Devière J (1995) Primary achalasia: analysis of endoscopic ultrasonography features with different instruments. Gastrointest Endosc Clin N Am 5(3):631–634

Edmundowicz SA (1995) Common bile duct stones. Gastrointest Endosc Clin N Am 5:817–824

Erickson RA, Chang KJ (1996) ERCP, EUS+ERCP, or MRCP+ERCP prior to laparoscopic cholecystectomy (LC): a cost-benefit analysis. Gastrointest Endosc 43:A83

Giovannini M, Seitz JF, Monges G, Perrier H, Rabbia I (1995) Fine-needle aspiration cytology guided by endoscopic ultrasonography: results in 141 patients. Endoscopy 27:171–177

Giovannini M (1995) Endoscopic ultrasonography with a curved array transducer: normal echoanatomy of retroperitoneum. Gastrointest Endosc Clin N Am 5(3):523–528

Goldberg BB, Hilpert PL, Burens PN et al (1990) Hepatic tumors: signal enhancement at Doppler us after intravenous injection of a contrast agent. Radiology 177:713–717

Gress F, Ciaccia D, Kiel J, Sherman S, Lehman G (1997) Endoscopic ultrasound guided celiac plexus block for management of pain due to chronic pancreatitis: a large single center experience. Gastrointest Endosc 45:A582

Gress F, Savides T, Cummings O, Sherman S, Lehman G, Zaidi S, Hawes R (1997) Radial scanning and linear array endosonography for staging pancreatic cancer: a prospective randomized comparison. Gastrointest Endosc 45(2):138–142

Gress FG, Hawes RH, Savides TJ, Ikenberry SO, Lehman GA (1997) Endoscopic ultrasound-guided fine-needle aspiration biopsy using linear array and radial scanning endosonography. Gastrointest Endosc 45(3):243–250

Grimm H, Hamper K, Binmoeller KF et al (1992) Enlarged lymph nodes: malignant or not? Endoscopy 24[Suppl 1]:320–323

Grimm H, Binmoeller KF et al (1992) Endosonography-guided drainage of a pancreatic pseudocyst. Gastrointest Endosc 38(2):170–171

Harada N, Wiersema M, Wiersema L (1997) Endosonography-guided celiac plexus neurolysis for abdominal pain: comparison of results in patients with chronic pancreatitis versus malignant disease. Gastrointest Endosc 45:A24

Hirooka Y, Naitoh Y, Goto H, Ito A, Taki T, Hayakawa T (1997) Usefulness of contrast-enhanced endoscopic ultrasonography with intravenous injection of sonicated serum albumin. Gastrointest Endosc 46:166–169

Hirooka Y, Goto H, Ito A et al (1998a) Contrast-enhanced endoscopic ultrasonography in pancreatic diseases: a preliminary study. Am J Gastroenterol 93:632–635

Hirooka Y, Naitoh Y, Goto H et al (1998b) Contrast-enhanced endoscopic ultrasonography in gallbladder diseases. Gastrointest Endosc 48:406–410

Hoffman BJ, Knapple W, Bhutani MS et al (1996) EUS-guided injection of botulinum toxin for achalasia. Gastrointest Endosc 43:A534

Imari Y, Sakamoto S, Shiomichi S, Isobe H, Ikeda M, Satoh M, Nawata H (1992) Hepatocellular carcinoma not detected with plain us: treatment with percutaneous ethanol injection under guidance with enhanced us. Radiology 185:497–500

Iwase H, Suga S, Morise K, Kuroiwa A, Yamaguchi T, Horiuchi Y (1995) Color Doppler endoscopic ultrasonography for the evaluation of gastric varices and endoscopic obliteration with cyanoacrylate glue. Gastrointest Endosc 41(2):150–154

Kato T, Tsukamoto Y, Naitoh Y, Mitake M, Hirooka Y, Furukawa T et al (1994) Ultrasonographic angiography in gallbladder diseases. Acta Radiol 35:606–613

Kato T, Tsukamoto Y, Naitoh Y et al (1995) Ultrasonographic and endoscopic ultrasonographic angiography in pancreatic mass lesions. Acta Radiol 36:381–387

Kawamoto K, Yamada Y, Furukawa N, Utsunomiya T, Haraguchi Y, Mizuguchi M, Oiwa T, Takano H, Masuda K (1997) Endoscopic submucosal tumorectomy for gastrointestinal submucosal tumors restricted to the submucosa: a new form of endoscopic minimal surgery. Gastrointest Endosc 46:311–3117

Klein AL, Bailey AS, Moura A et al (1993) Reliability of echocardiographic measurements of myocardial perfusion using commercially produced sonicated serum albumin (Albunex). J Am Coll Cardiol 22:1983–1993

Knox TA (1998) Endoscopic ultrasound. Diagnostic and therapeutic uses. Surg Endosc 12(8):1088–1090

Limberg B (1997) Sonographie des Gastrointestinaltraktes. Springer, Berlin Heidelberg New York

Matsuda Y , Yabuuchi I (1986) Hepatic tumors: us contrast enhancement with CO_2 microbubbles. Radiology 161:701–705

Mitake M, Nakazawa S, Naitoh Y, Kimoto E, Tsukamoto Y, Asai T (1990) Endoscopic ultrasonography in diagnosis of the extent of gallbladder carcinoma. Gastrointest Endosc 36:562–566

Nagamine N, Ueno N, Tomiyama T, Aizawa T, Tano S, Wada S, Suzuki T, Amagai K, Ono K, Kumakura Y, Hirasawa T, Ishino Y, Ido K, Kimura K (1998) A pilot study on modified endoscopic variceal ligation using endoscopic ultrasonography with color Doppler function. Am J Gastroenterol 93:150–155

Nickl NJ, Bhutani MS, Catalano M, Hoffman B, Hawes R, Chak A, Roubein LD, Kimmey M, Johnson M, Affronti J, Canto M, Sivak M, Boyce HW, Lightdale CJ, Stevens P, Schmitt C (1996) Clinical implications of endoscopic ultrasound: the American Endosonography Club Study. Gastrointest Endosc 44(4):371–377

Nomura N, Goto H, Niwa T et al (1999) Usefulness of contrast-enhanced endoscopic ultrasonography in the diagnosis of upper GI tract diseases. Gastrointest Endosc (in press)

Pavlick AC, Gerdes H, Portlock CS (1997) Endoscopic ultrasound in the evaluation of gastric small lymphocytic mucosa-associated lymphoid tumors. J Clin Oncol 15(5):1761–1766

Pedersen BH, Vilmann P, Folke K et al (1996) Endoscopic ultrasonography and real-time guided fine-needle aspiration biopsy of solid lesions of the mediastinum suspected of malignancy. Chest 110:539–544

Pitre J, Soubrane O, Palazzo L, Chapuis Y (1996) Endoscopic ultrasonography for the preoperative localization of insulinomas. Pancreas 13(1):55–60

Porter TR, Xie F, Kricsfeld A et al (1995) Noninvasive identification of acute myocardial ischemia and reperfuion with contrast ultrasound intravenous perfluoropropane-exposed sonicated dextrose albumin. J Am Coll Cardiol 26:33–40

Rice TW, Boyce GA, Sivak MV et al (1992) Esophageal carcinoma: esophageal ultrasound assessment of preoperative chemotherapy. Ann Thorac Surg 53:972–977

Rogers BM, Cicurel NJ et al (1975) Transgastric needle aspiration of pancreatic cysts through an endoscope. Gastrointestinal Endoscopy 21:132–133

Roesch T, Lightdale CJ, Botet JF et al (1992) Localization of pancreatic endocrine tumors by endoscopic ultrasonography. N Engl J Med 326:1721–1726

Roesch T, Lorenz R, Braig C et al (1991) Endoscopic ultrasound in pancreatic tumor diagnosis. Gastrointest Endosc 37:347–352

Roesch T (1995) Endoscopic ultrasonography in upper gastrointestinal submucosal tumors: a literature review. Gastrointest Endosc Clin N Am 5(3):609–614

Roesch T (1995) Endosonographic staging of esophageal cancer: a review of literature results. Gastrointest Endosc Clin N Am 5(3):537–547

Roesch T (1995) Endosonographic staging of gastric cancer: a review of literature results. Gastrointest Endosc Clin N Am 5(3):549–557

Roesch T (1995) Staging of pancreatic cancer. Analysis of literature results. Gastrointest Endosc Clin N Am 5(4):735–739

Roesch T, Classen M, in collaboration with Dittler, HJ (1992) Gastroenterologic endosonography. Thieme

Sahai AV, Hoffman BJ, Hawes RH (1998) Endoscopic ultrasound-guided hepaticogastrostomy to palliate obstructive jaundice: preliminary results in pigs. Gastrointest Endosc 47:AB37

Sahel, J (1990) Endoscopic cysto-enterostomy of cysts of chronic calcifying pancreatitis. Z Gastroenterol 28(3):170–172

Seifert H, Dietrich C et al (1999) Endosonography-guided one-step drainage of cystic lesions. Endoscopy (in press)

Snady H (1995) Vascular anatomy: how to identify the major retroperitoneal vessels. Gastrointest Endosc Clin N Am 5(3):497–506

Sugiyama M, Atomi Y, Kuroda A, Muto T, Wada N (1995) Large cholesterol polyps of the gallbladder: diagnosis by means of us and endoscopic us. Radiology 196:493–497

Taki T, Goto H, Naitoh Y et al (1997) Diagnosis of mucin-producing tumor of the pancreas with an intraductal ultrasonographic system. J Ultrasound Med 16:1–6

Ueno N, Tomiyama T, Tano S, Miyata Ta, Miyata To, Kimura K (1996) Contrast enhanced color Doppler ultrasonography in diagnosis of pancreatic tumor: two case reports. J Ultrasound Med 15:527–530

Vianna A, Peter CH, Moscoso G et al (1987) Normal venous circulation of the gastroesophageal junction: a route to understanding varices. Gastroenterology 93:876-8-89

Vilmann P, Hancke S, Henriksen FW, Jacobsen GK (1995) Endoscopic ultrasonography-guided fine-needle aspiration biopsy of lesions in the upper gastrointestinal tract. Gastrointest Endosc 41:230–235

Vilmann P, Hancke S, Henriksen FW, Jacobsen GK (1993) Endosonographically-guided fine needle aspiration biopsy of malignant lesions in the upper gastrointestinal tract. Endoscopy 25:523–527

Vilmann P, Hancke S (1996) A new biopsy handle instrument for endoscopic ultrasound-guided fine- needle aspiration biopsy. Gastrointest Endosc 43:238–242

Vilmann P, Jacobsen GK, Henriksen FW, Hancke S (1992) Endoscopic ultrasonography with guided fine needle aspiration biopsy in pancreatic disease. Gastrointest Endosc 38:172–173

Vilmann P (1998) Endoscopic ultrasonography with curved array transducer in diagnosis of cancer in and adjacent to the upper gastrointestinal tract. Scanning and guided fine needle aspiration biopsy. Munksgaard, Copenhagen

Vilmann P (1996) Endoscopic ultrasonography-guided fine needle aspiration biopsy of lymph nodes. Gastrointest Endosc 43 (2):24–29

Wegener M, Adamek RJ, Wedmann B, Pfaffenbach B (1994) Endosonographically guided fine-needle aspiration puncture of paraesophagogastric mass lesions: preliminary results. Endoscopy 26:586–591

Wiersema M, Wiersema L (1996) Endosonography guided celiac plexus neurolysis (EUS CPN) in patients with pain due to intra-abdominal malignancy (IAM) Gastrointest Endosc 43:A565

Wiersema MJ, Kochman ML, Cramer HM, Tao LC, Wiersema LM (1994) Endosonography-guided real-time fine-needle aspiration biopsy. Gastrointest Endosc 40:700–707

Wiersema MJ, Vilmann P, Giovannini M, Chang KJ, Wiersema LM (1997) Endosonography guided fine needle aspiration biopsy: diagnostic accuracy and complication assessment. Gastroenterology 112:1087–1095

Zimmer T, Stolzel U, Bader M, Koppenhagen K, Hamm B, Buhr H, Riecken EO, Wiedenmann B (1996) Endoscopic ultrasonography and somatostatin receptor scintigraphy in the preoperative localisation of insulinomas and gastrinomas. Gut 39(4):562–568

Abbreviations

ADV	adventitia		**LV**	left ventricle
AG	adrenal gland		**M**	mucosa
ANA	anastomosis		**MP**	muscularis propria
AO	aorta		**MV**	mitral valve
AV	aortic valve		**P**	pancreas
AZV	azygos vein		**PD**	pancreatic duct
B	balloon		**PL**	pleura
CBD	common bile duct		**PUA**	pulmonary artery
CON	confluence		**PUV**	pulmonary vein
CT	celiac trunk		**PV**	portal vein
DIA	diaphragm		**RA**	right atrium
DU	duodenum		**REA**	renal artery
ES	esophagus		**REV**	renal vein
EUS	endoscopic ultrasound		**RV**	right ventricle
FL	fluid		**S**	spleen
FNA	fine-needle aspiration biopsy		**SA**	splenic artery
FNI	fine-needle injection		**SE**	serosa
GB	gall bladder		**SI**	small intestine
GDA	gastroduodenal artery		**SM**	submucosa
HA	hepatic artery		**SMA**	superior mesenteric artery
HV	hepatic vein		**SMV**	superior mesenteric vein
ICV	inferior caval vein		**SP**	spine
K	kidney		**ST**	stomach
L	liver		**SV**	splenic vein
LA	left atrium		**TG**	thyroid gland
LU	lumen		**TR**	trachea
LN	lymph node		**TU**	tumor

Tumor Staging Classifications

Digestive System Tumors

Esophagus (TNM)

T1	Lamina propria, submucosa
T2	Muscularis propria
T3	Adventitia
T4	Adjacent structures
N1	Regional
M1	Distant metastasis

Tumor of lower thoracic esophagus

M1a	Celiac nodes
M1b	Other distant metastasis

Tumor of upper thoracic esophagus

M1a	Cervical nodes
M1b	Other distant metastasis

Tumor of midthoracic esophagus

M1b	Distant metastasis including nonregional lymph nodes

Stomach (TNM)

T1	Lamina propria, submucosa
T2	Muscularis propria, submucosa
T3	Penetrates serosa
T4	Adjacent structures
N1	1–6 nodes
N2	7–15 nodes
N3	>15 nodes

Gastrointestinal Malignant Lymphomas of the Mucosa-associated Tissue
(after Radaskiewicz)

EI	Gastrointestinal tract (localized) on the same side of the diaphragm
EI$_1$	Lamina propria, submucosa
EI$_2$	Muscularis propria, subserosa, serosa
EII	Gastrointestinal tract (localized) and regional lymph nodes on the same side of the diaphragm
EII$_1$	+ Regional lymph nodes
EII$_2$	+ Distant lymph nodes
EIII	Gastrointestinal tract (localized) and lymph nodes on both sides of the diaphragm
EIV	Disseminated organ involvement ± lymph nodes

Extrahepatic bile ducts (TNM)

T1	Ductal wall
T1a	Subepithelial connective tissue
T1b	Fibromuscular layer
T2	Perifibromuscular connective tissue
T3	Adjacent structures
N1	Hepatoduodenal ligament
N2	Other regional

Ampulla of Vater (TNM)

T1	Ampulla or sphincter of Oddi
T2	Duodenal wall
T3	Pancreas ≤ 2 cm
T4	Pancreas >2 cm, other organs
N1	Regional

Pancreas (TNM)

T1	Limited to the pancreas ≤ 2 cm
T2	Limited to the pancreas >2 cm
T3	Duodenum, bile duct, peripancreatic tissues
T4	Stomach, spleen, colon, large vessels
N1	Regional
N1a	Single node
N1b	Multiple nodes

Lung carcinomas

Lung (TNM)

TX	Positive cytology
T1	≤ 3 cm
T2	> 3 cm, main bronchus 2 cm from carina, invades visceral pleura, partial atelectasis
T3	Chest wall, diaphragm, pericardium, mediastinal pleura, main bronchus < 2 cm from carina, total atelectasis
T4	Mediastinum, heart, great vessels, carina, trachea, esophagus, vertebra; separate nodules in same lobe, malignant effusion
N1	Ipsilateral peribronchial, ipsilateral hilar
N2	Ipsilateral mediastinal, subcarinal
N3	Contalateral mediastinal or hilar, scalene or supraclavicular
M1	Includes separate nodule in different lobe

Subject Index